Heat Illness and Critical Care

Edited by Nissar Shaikh

Published in London, United Kingdom

Heat Illness and Critical Care
http://dx.doi.org/10.5772/intechopen.104339
Edited by Nissar Shaikh

Contributors
Anna Olegovna Petrova, Darya V. Ryzhkova, Elena G. Potemkina, Eleonora T. Nazaralieva, Galal Alessai, Gamal Al-Ameri, Hoang Thanh Tuan, Hongyan Cai, Hossam Algallie, Irina Alexandrovna Savvina, Ivayla I. Geneva, Jiaying Yu, Konstantin E. Lebedev, Kristina M. Bykova, Lixing Huang, Mohammed Helboob, Mubarak Alhatemi, Muhammad Zubair, Natalya V. Dryagina, Nissar Shaikh, Qiu Li, Rumeel Ahmad Bhutta, Sanja Stankovic, Sengkwan Choi, Umme Nashrah, Wael Khalaf, Waleed Salem, Youyu Zhang, Zia Mahmood Awan

First published in London, United Kingdom, 2024 by IntechOpen
IntechOpen is the global imprint of INTECHOPEN LIMITED, registered in England and Wales, registration number: 11086078, 167-169 Great Portland Street, London, W1W 5PF, United Kingdom

British Library Cataloguing-in-Publication Data
A catalogue record for this book is available from the British Library

Additional hard and PDF copies can be obtained from orders@intechopen.com

Heat Illness and Critical Care
Edited by Nissar Shaikh
p. cm.
Print ISBN 978-1-83768-903-3
Online ISBN 978-1-83768-904-0
eBook (PDF) ISBN 978-1-83768-905-7

For EU product safety concerns:
IN TECH d.o.o., Prolaz Marije Krucifikse Kozulić 3, 51000 Rijeka, Croatia, info@intechopen.com or visit our website at intechopen.com.

Meet the editor

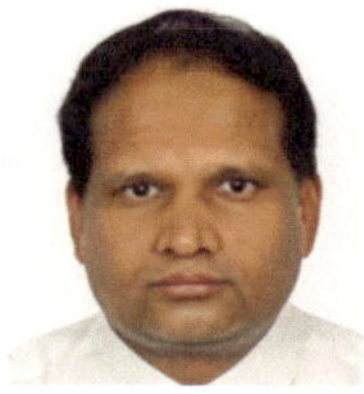

Dr. Nissar Shaikh, MD, EDIC, DID, FCCM, is a senior intensive care consultant and surgical intensive care fellowship director at Hamad Medical Corporation, Qatar. He is an associate professor at Qatar University College of Medicine and assistant professor at Weill Cornell Medicine–Qatar and an associate professor at the College of Medicine, Qatar University. Dr. Nissar has made numerous oral and poster presentations at national and international conferences. He has 200 peer-reviewed publications in critical and acute care to his credit as well as four books and 34 book chapters. He has won three prestigious awards for distinguished services from Hamad Medical Corporation.

Contents

Preface

Heat Illness and Critical Care describes the management of acute and critically ill patients due to exposure to the heat. It discusses important topics in acute care and diagnosis of heat-related illnesses. Chapters address professionalism and teamwork in the management of heat-related illnesses. This book is a useful resource for emergency and acute care physicians, EMS staff, and acute and critical care nurses. We are thankful to Ms. Kristina Kardum Cvitan for her continuous help at all stages of the publication process. I am indebted and thankful to Dr. Firdos for her support and encouragement during the editing process. I am grateful for the patience and cooperation of my daughters Dr. Amara and Dr. Jaza. Finally, I wish to acknowledge the participating authors for their valuable contributions.

Nissar Shaikh
Surgical Intensive Care Unit,
Hamad Medical Corporation,
Doha, Qatar

Chapter 1

Introductory Chapter: Heat-Related Illness – Need for Awareness, Attention and Research

Nissar Shaikh

1. Introduction

Heat-related illnesses are increasing rapidly and significantly. In the past two decades, there has been more than 50% increase in heat-related illness, morbidity and mortality particularly in elderly patients. The increase in heat-related illness is closely related to global warming and extreme heat events from east to the west. This increase in heat-related illness is causing a rise in intensive care therapy utilization, hospitalization with simoultenousely significant increase in global health burden and larger economic impact [1].

With further expected rise in global temperature by mid-century will result in a fivefold rise in extreme heat events and instead of occurring once in 50 years, they will increase by 14 times [1]. Hence it is of the utmost importance to be aware of these heat-related illnesses, their management and prevention.

2. Risk factors

The risk of these heat-related illnesses increases significantly when exposed to the extremes of temperature particularly in susceptible individuals such as extremes of age, pregnant and patients with multiple comorbidities. The environmental risk for occurrence of these illnesses ranges from poor socioeconomical status to the limited labor protection and accesses to health care [1].

3. Management

Heat stroke is the most serious of the heat-related illnesses, and it is a medical emergency, classified into exertional which typically occurs in healthy persons and classic heat stroke which occurs in patients with risk factors and comorbidities. In heat stroke, there are abnormalities in dissipation of the excessive body heat leading to the cellular and organ dysfunction including damage to the gastrointestinal system causing endotoxemia and triggering profound systemic inflammatory response syndrome causing further cellular and organ injury. The triad of heat stroke is elevated body temperature (40°C), intravascular coagulopathy and central nervous system disturbances [2].

IntechOpen

The other heat-related illnesses are heat exhaustion and heat cramps, edema and rash are mild to moderate disease (**Figure 1**). Apart from the above heat-related illnesses, the exposure to extremes of heat with elevated body temperature leads to exacerbation of heart disease, ischemic stroke, respiratory tract infections, kidney diseases, psychiatric disorder and preterm labor and delivery [3].

Heat stroke being a clinical and medical emergency has to be differentiated, and diagnosed quickly with early treatment as it is essential to prevent neurological complications with increased morbidity and mortality.

The most important point in the diagnosis of heat stroke is an accurate and timely measurement of the core body temperature. Usually, the rectal temperature is measured. The signs and symptoms of these heat-related illnesses depend on severity, heat stroke is typically diagnosed by the presence of triad of history of exposure to higher temperature, hyperthermia and neurological dysfunction. The presence of neurological abnormalities differentiates heat stroke from other heat-related illnesses. Heat stroke manifests in three phases, earlier diagnosis is better for clinical outcome. The acute phase is characterized by hyperthermia and neurological dysfunction, the 2nd phase occurs from 24 to 48 hours and is manifested by coagulopathy and enzymatic disorders. The late phase occurs 96 hours or longer after exposure to the extreme temperature and is manifested by multiple organ dysfunction [2].

The treatment of mild to moderate heat-related illnesses is mainly symptomatic and supportive (**Figure 1**) whereas the heat stroke patients should be managed by a multidisciplinary team, in intensive care therapy settings. The corner stone in the treatment of heat stroke is the rapid cooling and achieving the targeted temperature

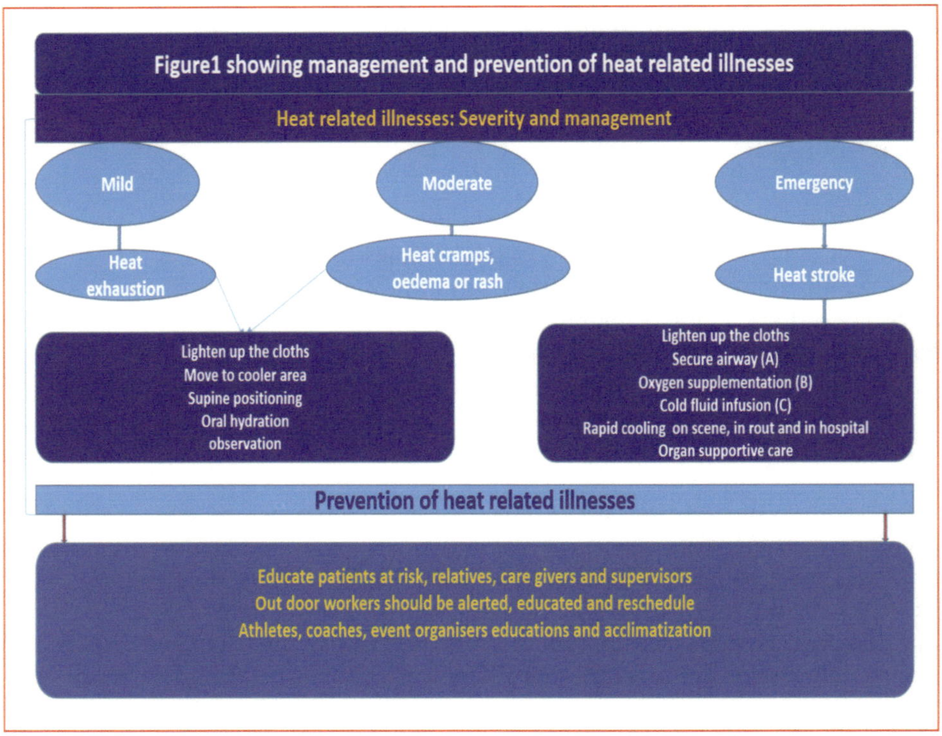

Figure 1.
Showing management and prevention of heat related illnesses.

(frequently around 38°C) within 30 minutes by rapid blood, esophageal or surface cooling methods along with taking care of airway, breathing and circulation. The pharmacological interventions are not very effective and causes adverse effects. Further in the care of these patients will be organ-supportive therapy [3].

4. Further research

Research and high-quality studies are limited and require advanced knowledge and research regarding the effective rate and method of rapid cooling, when to stop cooling as well as about the medications to be used in heat stroke patients. Further research and reports are required about the impact of heat wave awareness and the use of early warning systems and alerts [4, 5]. Although there are excellent guidelines for the management of heat-related illnesses, more protocols and guidelines are needed in other different settings occurrence of this disease [6].

5. Prevention

Heat-related illnesses are preventable (**Figure 1**). Hence all the efforts should be taken for identifying patients at risk, educating not only patients but their relatives, care givers, social workers about awareness, preventive measures and seeking early health care. Not only athletes, but spectators, administrators, event organizers, coaches, staff should be educated about heat exposure and heat-related illnesses, and athletes should be acclimatized in advance for shorter training sessions for extreme heat exposure [7]. About 75% of fatalities at work in the extreme of temperature occur during the first week. Outdoor workers and their supervisors should also be educated and made aware about day to day extreme temperatures and risk of heat-related illnesses and encourage them to drink water frequently, remove extra clothes and equipment. We recommend in extreme summer days, outdoor construction and other work should be in the early hours of day and in the evening and to rest in the afternoon when the temperature is maximum. Few countries follow the rule of 20%, in the first week of work in extreme summer, worker should work only 20% of the shift and in further weeks also do 20% work of the day till acclimatize to the extremely warm weather (**Figure 1**) [5].

Author details

Nissar Shaikh
Surgical Intensive Care Unit: Hamad Medical Corporation, Doha, Qatar

*Address all correspondence to: nissatfirdous99@gmail.com

References

[1] Sorensen C, Hess J. Treatment and prevention of heat related illness. The New England Journal of Medicine. 2022;**387**:1404-1413

[2] Epstein Y, Yanovich BK. Heat stroke. The New England Journal of Medicine. 2019;**380**:2449-2459

[3] Basu R, Pearson MB, Broadwins R, Green R. The effects of high ambient temperature on emergency room visits. Epidemiology. 2012;**23**:813-820

[4] Dwyer IJ, Barry SJE, Megiddo I, White CJ. Evaluations of heat action plans for reducing the health impacts of extreme heat: Methodological developments (2012-2021) and remaining challenges. International Journal of Biometeorology. 2022;**66**(9):1915-1927

[5] Gubernot DM, Anderson GB, Hunting KL. The epidemiology of occupational heat exposure in the United States: A review of the literature and assessment of research needs in a changing climate. International Journal of Biometeorology. 2014;**58**(8):1779-1788

[6] Almuzaini Y, Abdulmalek N, Ghallab S, Mushi A, Yassin Y, Yezli S, et al. Adherence of healthcare workers to saudi management guidelines of heat-related illnesses during hajj pilgrimage. International Journal of Environmental Research and Public Health. 28 Jan 2021;**18**(3):1156

[7] Roberts WO, Armstrong LE, Sawka MN, Yeargin SW, Heled Y, O'Connor FG. ACSM expert consensus statement on exertional heat illness: Recognition, management, and return to activity. Current Sports Medicine Reports. 2021;**20**(9):470-484

Chapter 2

Acute Management of Heat Stroke: Facts and Figures

Gamal Al-Ameri, Waleed Salem, Galal Alessai, Mohammed Hellboob, Mubarak Alhatemi, Umme Nashrah and Nissar Shaikh

Abstract

Heat-related illnesses range from heat exhaustion to heat stroke. Heat stroke is a life-threatening medical emergency causing multiple organ dysfunction that if not treated, can be fatal. It is a severe heat illness with a body temperature of more than 40^0c and organ dysfunction. Epidemiology of heat stroke varies depending on geographic location, and reported incidences range from 1.98 to 2.89/100000 per year. Heat stroke is classified as exertional or non-exertional. Pathophysiology is exposure to higher temperatures with impaired thermoregulation. Patients will present with high core body temperature; tachypnea, tachycardia, and hypotension may be present. The manifestations of organ dysfunction range from coagulopathy to altered levels of consciousness, and pulmonary edema. Accurate core body temperature measurement with clinical manifestations will diagnose the heat stroke. Early diagnosis, earlier temperature management, and organ supportive care are essential.

Keywords: core body temperature, emergency, heat stroke, temperature management, organ supportive care

1. Introduction

Heat-related illness is a spectrum of conditions that severely increase from heat exhaustion and heat injury to life-threatening emergency called heat stroke. The manifestation of heat stroke ranges from delirium to seizures. Heat stroke, or sunstroke, is a life-threatening emergency. It is a severe heat illness that increases body temperature to more than 40°C (104 F), heat stroke causes more than 600 deaths per year in the US [1].

2. Epidemiology

In the United States, from 2006 to 2010, it was reported to have caused at least 3332 deaths. Heat stroke mortality is correlated with the degree of body temperature elevation, time of initiation of cooling, and number of organs affected [2].

Various aspects can affect the incidence of heat stroke, including gender, age, geographic location, and occupation. Heat stroke is higher in females, with a female-to-male ratio of up to 2.89 versus 0.98–1.98 per 1000 person-years [3].

Heat stroke has different rates of occurrence in different geographic areas. During the European heat wave in 2022, thousands of people died due to heat stroke. Heat stroke mortality is expected to rise by 2.5 times by 2050 [3].

3. Classification and definition

Bouchama's definition is the most commonly accepted for heat stroke, and it is a rise in core body temperature of more than 40°C with hot, dry skin and central nervous system abnormalities. Another alternative definition of heat stroke is the hyperthermia associated with SIRS (Systemic Inflammatory Response Syndrome), which causes multiple organ dysfunction and mainly central nervous system dysfunction [4].

The JAAM heat stroke committee (Japanese Association for Acute Medicine) heat stroke committee, after analysis of the data collected by the working group, modified the heat stroke definition. Heat stroke is defined as patients exposed to high environmental temperatures who meet one or more of the following criteria [5]:

1. Glasgow Coma Scale (GCS) score of $\leq$14,

2. Creatinine or total bilirubin levels of $\geq$1.2 mg/dL,

3. JAAM DIC score of $\geq$4.

4. Classification

Heat stroke is typically classified into two groups depending upon the presence or absence of exertion [4, 5].

1. The exertion of heat stroke occurs in healthy individuals performing rigorous physical activity in higher environmental temperatures.

2. The non-exertional heat stroke develops during minimal physical activity in elderly persons with comorbidities including hypertension, diabetes mellitus, obesity, renal and cardiac disease, or alcoholism.

Non-exertional or classic heat stroke occurs in individuals at extremes of age, elderly over 70, or children in the vehicle. The main issue in this type of heat stroke is an anatomical or physiological predisposition or the patient's comorbidities, all of which impair thermoregulation, prevent removal from a hot environment, or interfere with access to hydration or attempts at cooling. Prescribed or recreational medication, anticholinergics, beta-blockers or diuretics, and cocaine and alcohol, respectively, also contribute to non-exertional heat stroke. Exertional heat stroke occurs when a healthy individual heavily exercises at a higher ambient temperature.

5. Pathophysiology

5.1 Thermoregulation

The human body maintains a temperature of 37 C, through convection, conduction, radiation, and vaporization, which are controlled by the hypothalamus. In cases of an increase in body temperature, the sympathetic system is activated, causing cutaneous vasodilation and thermal sweating. These also cause a loss of intravascular volume and salt, leading to dehydration. Increased severity causes further loss of water with salt, leading to impaired thermoregulation and reduction of visceral blood volume with shunting to the skin and muscles, resulting in organ dysfunction (above). In response to stress, body cells generate heat stroke proteins (HSP). An increase in HSP is essential for heat tolerance, and overexpression of HSP protects against organ impairment.

The increase in body temperature causes intestinal mucosal injury, and the release of endotoxins and proinflammatory mediators interleukins 1 and 6 from muscles to the systemic circulation, these chemicals leucocytes and endothelial cells, and the release of various cytokines and HMGB (high mobility group box 1 protein), all in combination stimulate SIRS (systemic inflammatory response syndrome) (**Figure 1**) [5].

The heat stroke thus generates inflammatory and coagulopathy responses; the direct effect of heat also causes endothelial injury and generates microthromboses, leading to a disseminated intravascular coagulation (DIC) response.

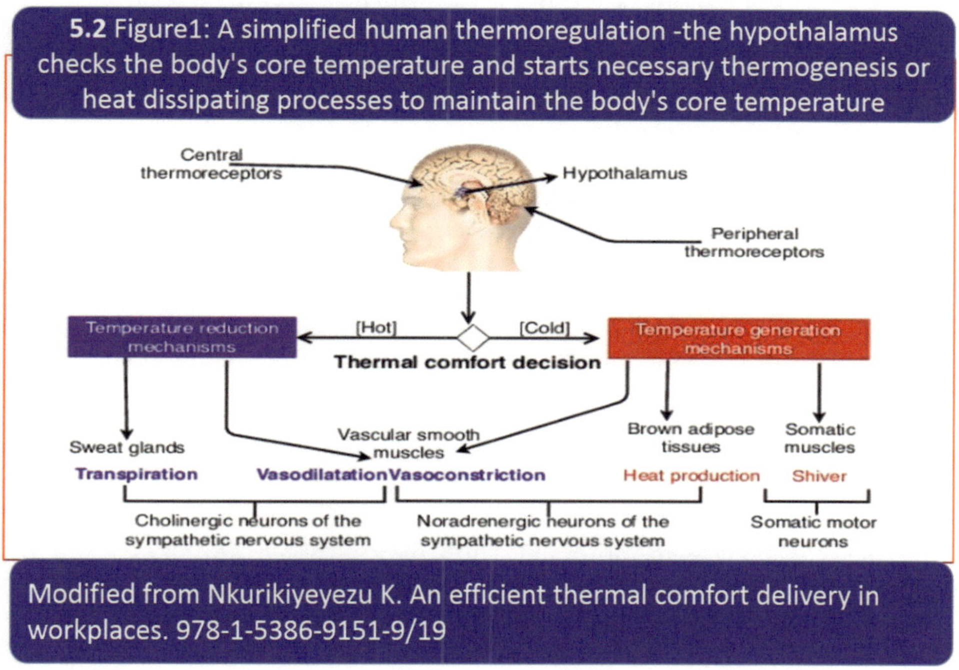

Figure 1.
A simplified human thermoregulation –the hypothalamus checks the body's core temperature and starts necessary thermogenesis or heat dissipating processes to maintain the body's core temperature. Modified from Nkurikiyeyezu K. An efficient thermal comfort delivery in workplaces. 978-1-5386-9151-9/19.

Diuretic therapy
Elderly (> 70 years)
Cardiac disease
Oncological disorders
Core body temperature > 40°C
Hypotension
Hypertension
Renal dysfunctions
Coagulopathy
Requirement of vasopressors
Decrease conscious level
hypoxia
No air cooling,

Table 1.
Prognostic factors.

6. Prognostic factors

Table 1 shows prognostic factors in patients with heat stroke. These factors increase mortality and morbidity.

7. Risk factors for heat stroke

The factors that increase the chances of a classic heat stroke are age, obesity, poor physical condition, lack of acclimatization, no air conditioning, and social isolation. Other risk factors are the use of illicit drugs, recreational drugs, and comorbidities such as cardiovascular disease and diabetes mellitus.

The factors associated with increased mortality and morbidity in heat-exertion patients are the degree of temperature elevation and the number of organ dysfunction [1, 5].

8. Clinical presentation

Elevated core body temperature and central nervous system disorder are diagnostic presentations of heat stroke.

With increased body temperature or hyperthermia, there will be tachycardia, tachypnea, wide pulse pressure, and hypotension mostly due to dehydration. Organ dysfunction can manifest as noncardiogenic pulmonary edema with crepitation and desaturation.

If coagulopathy is severe will be skin rashes, petechiae, and ecchymosis, the neurological dysfunction will be manifested by an altered level of consciousness, speech distortion, agitation and irritability, seizure, or coma [6].

9. Diagnosis

A missed diagnosis of heat stroke increases mortality and morbidity. Accurate measurement of core body temperature is essential in these patients. The X-ray chest may show diffuse infiltrates and signs of pulmonary edema. ECG may show different changes, from dysrhythmias to ST segment changes [1, 4].

CBC (complete blood count), renal function, coagulation parameters, and serum urinary electrolytes may be deranged. Usually, liver function takes a day or two to be deranged.

10. Management

Early diagnosis, quicker cooling, correction of electrolyte abnormalities, and supportive care are essential for a better patient outcome.

Depending on the patient's level of consciousness, if the patient is still able to obey commands, oxygen supplementation via face mask or nasal cannula should be enough. If the patient has lower GCS and cannot protect the airway, intubation, and mechanical ventilation are mandatory.

Hypotension or shock management should be guided in critically ill patients with the use of novel tools for hemodynamic monitoring and the use of point-of-care ultrasound technologies.

These patients, if still hypotensive after resuscitation, may require vasopressors and inotropes. Cooling with temperature monitoring. Rapid cooling with accurate core body temperature monitoring is essential for patients with heat stroke.

Evaporative and connective cooling are found to have a better outcome, as they are effective maneuver and easy to perform.

Evaporative and connective cooling are performed with a spray of a moist tube of warm water and using fans to blow air over the moist skin of a naked patient.

The technique may require sedation with shorter-acting agents, particularly if patients are irritable or have altered mental status.

Immersing these patients in ice water is also a rapid, noninvasive method of cooling patients. Those patients are immersed, and it is difficult to have a venous cannula. Another alternative is to place the patient on a porous stretcher positioned on top of a tub of ice water and have paramedical staff continuously pour ice water from the bath onto to patient and manage the major muscular area [7]. Here, we can better monitor patients and have intravascular accesses.

Otherwise continuously applying ice to the axilla, neck, and groin will also help in cooling.

More invasive is peritoneal and pleural cold water. Continuous lavage is an alternative but is invasive, and one has to be careful in patients with coagulopathy. More recently, intranasal cooling was also used in those patients [7].

Pharmacological therapy and alcohol sponges should be avoided. Alcohol may get absorbed by dilated skin vessels and may cause toxicity, whereas those anti pyritic medications, aspirin, and paracetamol are not useful in heat stroke patients as the mechanism does not involve a change in the hypothalamic set point. These may cause adverse effects on the liver [5, 7, 8].

All these patients' temperatures should be monitored continuously and accurately, either by rectal or oropharyngeal temperature monitoring.

Cooling measures should be stopped once a temperature of 38 or 39C is achieved in order to reduce the iatrogenic hypothermia [8].

11. Organ dysfunction and its management

Heat stroke can cause multiple organ dysfunction. We will describe the heat stroke causing multiple organ dysfunction in system-wise order.

11.1 Respiratory dysfunction

Heat stroke patients can have aspiration pneumonia, bronchospasm, non-cardiogenic pulmonary edema, pneumonitis, pulmonary hemorrhage, and infection. Invasive ventilation with endotracheal intubation enables protection of the airway and management of increased metabolic demand through oxygen supplement and increased minute ventilation [9].

11.2 Cardiac dysfunction

Heat stroke can cause acute cardiac decompensation and myocardial injury, with reversible cardiac biomarkers elevation. Cardiac dysfunction and tachyarrhythmias respond well to cooling, hence anti-arrhythmics are seldom necessary, and electric cardioversion should be avoided until cooling is achieved unless necessary to treat VF (ventricular fibrillation) or PVT (pulseless ventricular tachycardia) [9].

11.3 Hypotension

Hypotension in these patients is due to volume depletion, vasodilation, and cardiac dysfunction, therapy is isotonic or crystalloid fluid resuscitation, and alpha-adrenergic medication impairs cooling and should be avoided [9].

11.4 CNS dysfunction

Cerebral edema and seizure are frequent CNS complications in heat stroke patients.

A variety of cerebrovascular disorders ranging from neuropathies, Gillian-Barre Syndrome, and Parkinsonism are reported in heat stroke patients [10].

Standard anticonvulsant and anti-edema measures can be followed in these patients with continuous EEG monitoring.

11.5 Rhabdomyolysis

Rhabdomyolysis is frequent in heat stroke patients, and can be typically managed by hydration-forced diuresis and electrolyte management.

11.6 Acute kidney injury

Heat stroke patients will have AKI due to severe dehydration, or rhabdomyolysis. Serum electrolyte and renal functions should be monitored regularly and depending on AKI severity, may require renal replacement therapy.

11.7 Hepatic injury

The liver function should be monitored in patients with heat stroke, liver injury in these patients is self-limited but can progress to hepatic failure and require transplant [11].

11.8 Disseminated intravascular coagulation (DIC)

DIC is more frequent in patients with heat stroke during the initial 72 hours. All these should be monitored with traditional coagulation parameters (PT, aPTT, INR, fibrinogen, D-Dimer) and state of art management such as ROTEM. If required, DIC can be treated with the replacement of clotting factors, fresh frozen plasma, or prothrombin complex.

12. Mortality and outcome

Heat stroke patients' outcomes depend on early diagnosis, early cooling, and prevention and treatment of organ dysfunction. These patients are at higher risk compared to the control group for myocardial ischemia, kidney injury, and ischemic stroke in the long term [12].

In these patients regardless of a number of organ dysfunction, the heat stroke survivors will have long-term functional and neurological disorders and impairment, with reported 28-day mortality of 58% and 2-year mortality of 71% [13].

13. Conclusion

Heat stork is a severe temperature-related illness, an acute medical illness, and a medical emergency. It is more common in females than males. Heat stroke is defined as a core body temperature of more than 40^0c with hot and dry skin associated with central nervous system dysfunction. Typically divided into exertional and non-exertional heat stroke. Heat stroke generates a systemic inflammatory and coagulopathy response in combination with heat injury causes organ dysfunctions. Diagnosed with raised body temperature with clinical manifestation and signs and symptoms of organ dysfunction or failure.

In the management of heat stroke ABCDE approach should be followed. Early body temperature management in combination with organ-supportive care will improve the clinical outcome. The mortality from heat stroke ranges from 58 to 71%.

Author details

Gamal Al-Ameri[1*], Waleed Salem[2], Galal Alessai[2], Mohammed Hellboob[2], Mubarak Alhatemi[2], Umme Nashrah[3] and Nissar Shaikh[1]

1 Surgical Intensive Care, Hamad Medical Corporation, Doha, Qatar

2 Accident and Emergency Department, Hamad Medical Corporation, Doha, Qatar

3 Deccan College of Medical Science, Hyderabad, India

*Address all correspondence to: drgamalabdulrahman@gmail.com

References

[1] Gaudio FG, Grissom CK. Cooling methods in heat stroke. The Journal of Emergency Medicine. 2016;**50**(4):607-616

[2] Pease S, Bouadma L, Kermarrec N, Schortgen F, Régnier B, Wolff M. Early organ dysfunction course, cooling time and outcome in classic heatstroke. Intensive Care Medicine. 2009;**35**(8):1454-1458

[3] Alele F, Malau-Aduli B, Malau-Aduli A, Crowe M. Systematic review of gender differences in the epidemiology and risk factors of exertional heat illness and heat tolerance in the armed forces. BMJ Open. 2020;**10**(4):e03182

[4] Bouchama A, Knochel JP. Heat stroke. The New England Journal of Medicine. 2002;**346**(25):1978-1978

[5] Singh RK, Baronia AK, Sahoo JN, Sharma S, Naval R, Pandey CM, et al. Prospective comparison of new Japanese Association for Acute Medicine (JAAM) DIC and International Society of Thrombosis and Hemostasis (ISTH) DIC score in critically ill septic patients. Thrombosis Research. 2012;**129**:e119-e125

[6] Epstein Y et al. Heat stroke. The New England Journal of Medicine. 2019;**380**(25):2449

[7] Manegold R et al. Effective intranasal cooling in an 80-year-old patient with heatstroke. American Journal of Emergency Medicine. 2020;**38**(11):2488

[8] Tek D, Olshaker JS. Heat illness. Emergency Medicine Clinics of North America. 1992;**10**(2):299-231

[9] Varghese GM, John G, Thomas K, Abraham OC, Mathai D. Predictors of multi-organ dysfunction in heatstroke. Emergency Medicine Journal. 2005;**22**(3):185-187

[10] Biary N, Madkour MM, Sharif H. Post-heatstroke parkinsonism and cerebellar dysfunction. Clinical Neurology and Neurosurgery. 1995;**97**(1):55-57

[11] Martínez-Insfran LA, Alconchel F, Ramírez P. Liver transplantation for fulminant hepatic failure due to heat stroke: A case report. Transplantation Proceedings. 2019;**51**(1):87-89

[12] Wang J-C, Chien W-C, Chu P. The association between heat stroke and subsequent cardiovascular diseases. PLoS One. 2019;**14**(2):e0211386

[13] Argaud L, Ferry T, Le Q-H, Marfisi A. Short- and long-term outcomes of heatstroke following the 2003 heat wave in Lyon, France. Archives of Internal Medicine. 2007;**167**(20):2177-2183

Chapter 3

Perioperative Thyroid Storm: A Medical and Surgical Emergency

Mohammad Zubair, Wael Khalaf, Zia Awan, Hossam Algallie, Nissar Shaikh and Gamal Al-Ameri

Abstract

Thyroid storm is rare, acute medical endocrine emergency. It is aggressive manifestation of the hyperthyroid state. If delayed or not treated can be fatal or cause severe disabilities. Historically thyroid storm was a common complication of toxic goiter and goiter surgery but recently more common in hyperthyroidism patients with acute illness or surgical intervention and inadequately treated hyperthyroid patients. There is usually precipitating factor that lead to thyroid storm, such as emergency surgery, extreme stress, or acute severe illness. Clinical manifestations involve major body organ dysfunctions and range from fever, dysrhythmias, heart failure, vomiting, diarrhea, jaundice, and convulsions to coma. The pathophysiology of thyroid storm is organ dysfunction due to excessive thyroid hormones. Thyroid storm is diagnosed by clinical presentation, Electrocardiogram (ECG), chest X-ray findings and thyroid point of care ultrasound (POCUS), and the scoring systems. Management should be started without delay. Apart from supportive care airway, breathing, circulation, and disability (ABCD) approach and antithyroid medications should be administered. Delay in management will increase morbidity and mortality. Initially, propylthiouracil (PTU), beta-blocker, iodine, steroids, and bile chelating agent are the treatment. The thyroid mortality ranges from 20 to 30%.

Keywords: thyroid storm, fatal, precipitating factors, thyroxine T3 and T4 toxicosis, arrhythmias, fever, multiorgan dysfunctions, beta-blockers, iodine, steroid, bile chelating agents

1. Introduction

Thyroid storm is an acute and rare life-threatening clinical condition, complicated manifestation of severe hyperthyroidism, with multiple organ involvement. It was described in 1926 that thyroid storm had high morbidity and mortality, despite advancement in medical sciences. Hence it is essential to recognize this life-threatening syndrome early and manage it earlier to improve patient's outcome. It is equally important that acute care physicians, surgeons and general practitioners, intensivists, and paramedical staffs are accustomed to the presentation and management of this rare endocrine disease [1].

2. Epidemiology

Thyroid storm is a rare presentation of hyperthyroidism. It accounts for 1–2% of hyperthyroidism admission. The reported incidence of thyroid storm in United States of America (USA) ranges from 0.5 to 0.7% cases/100,000 of normal population per year, where it is 4.8 to 5.6% /100,000 hospitalized patients [2]. The incidence of thyroid storm from Japan is 0.2/100,000 population per year. The thyroid storm patients were younger (42–43 years) and male to female ratio was 1:3 [3].

3. Precipitating factors

There are number of factors that may lead to the thyroid storm [4], described in the following **Table 1**.

The addition to above mentioned precipitating factors for thyroid storm, the severe emotional distress, and extreme stress can also lead to thyroid storm in hyperthyroid patients.

3.1 Pathophysiology of thyroid storm

Thyroid storm pathophysiology is summarized in **Figure 1**.

Several theories are proposed for thyroid storm. A precipitating factor is always required to initiate thyroid storm, the most accepted hypothesis is that rapid, sudden increase in thyroid hormone levels, thus free hormones released from the protein-bound hormones, causing sudden increase in body metabolism, thus causing an exaggerated signs and manifestations of hyperthyroidism with multiple organs dysfunction (**Table 1**).

The histopathologic findings depend upon the etiology of thyroid storm, if it is due to Graves' disease goiter, the histopathology will show diffuse follicular hyperplasia along with increased receptor antibodies with increased vascularity. If thyroid storm is due to malignancy, the histopathology will reveal ruptured follicles with malignant cells inhibition with disturbs of thyroid cells [5].

Sudden stoppage of antithyroid medications
Trauma/Thyroid surgeries
Acute illness (Myocardial infarction, cerebrovascular accidents, sepsis, emergency surgery)
Parturition
iodinated contrast
Burns
Amiodarone, salicylate and anesthetics
Hyperemesis gravidarum
Radiation exposure

Table 1.
Precipitating factors for the thyroid storm.

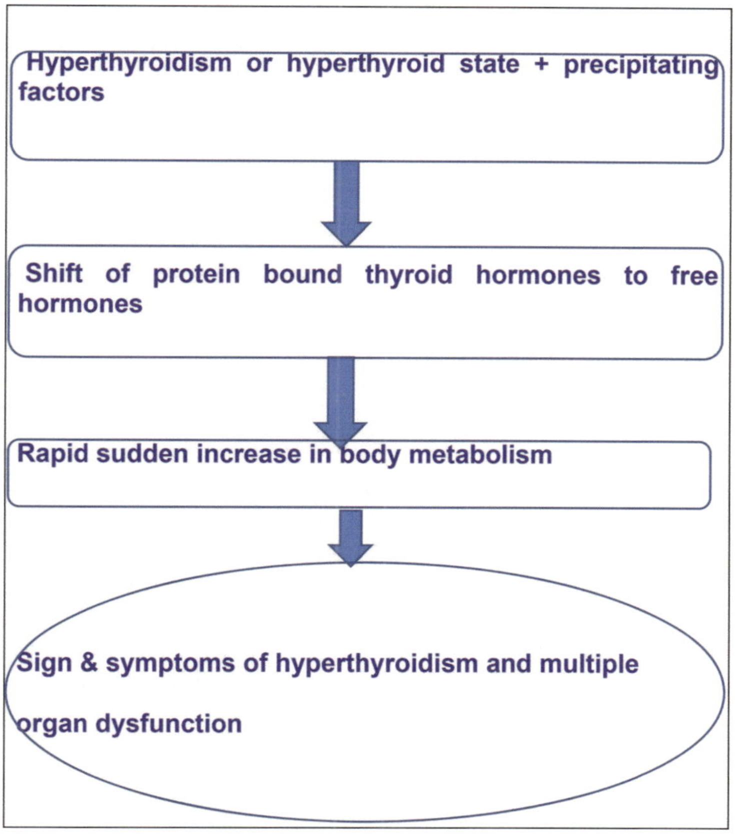

Figure 1.
Pathophysiology of thyroid storm.

3.2 Etiology

The thyroid storm commonly occurs in Graves' disease, toxic adenoma, and the multi-nodular toxic goiter. The exact etiology of thyroid storm is not known, there will be always a precipitating factor and the extremes of stress concurrent, systemic acute illness such as sepsis or increasing incidence with emergency surgery.

3.3 Clinical presentation

Patient thyroid storm will have exaggerated hyperthyroidism signs and symptoms. Fever, tachycardia, tachyarrhythmias and heart failure, central nervous system (CNS), and Gastrointestinal (GI) manifestations are frequent. The CNS manifestations will be agitation, delirium, anxiety, and coma. The GI symptoms are nausea, vomiting, diarrhea, intestinal obstruction, and hepatic failure. Examinations will reveal orbitopathy, goiter, hand tremors, moist and warm skin, and jaundice [6].

Common signs and symptoms are summarized in the following **Table 2**.

Thyrotoxicosis	Thyroid storm
Heat intolerance and diaphoresis	Hyperpyrexia, temperature > 106F with dehydration
Sinus tachycardia Heart rate 100 to 140/minute	Heart rate > 140 Tachyarrhythmias Hypertension Congestive heart failure
Diarrhea, increased appetite with weight loss	Nausea, vomiting, diarrhea, jaundice
Anxiety, restlessness	Agitation, confusion, delirium, seizures, and coma

Table 2.
Common signs and symptoms for thyrotoxicosis and thyroid storm.

3.4 Diagnosis

Thyroid storm should be suspected from clinical presentations in hyperthyroidism or suspected hyperthyroidism patients. Laboratory workup will show low thyroid stimulating hormone (TSH) and high T3/T4 levels. Patient will have hyperglycemia, hypercalcemia, leukocytosis, and abnormal liver function test. Various scoring systems for the diagnosis of thyroid storm are described in **Tables 3** and **4** [8].

According to the Japanese thyroid association (JTA), it is essential to diagnose thyroid storm by the elevated free T3 or T4 with one CNS manifestation and pulmonary

Burch–Wartofsky Point Scale (BWPS)	
Variables	**Points**
Temperature	5 points per 1 °F above 99°F (maximum 30 points)
CNS dysfunction: Agitation Delirium/lethargy Seizure/coma	10 points 20 points 30 points
Tachycardia 99–109/minute 110–119/minute 120–129/minute 130–139/minute >140/minute	5 points 10 points 15 points 20 points 25 points
Arterial fibrillation	10 points
GI dysfunction Vomiting/diarrhea Jaundice	10 points 20 points
Heart failure Pedal edema bi-basilar rales pulmonary edema	5 points 10 points 15 points
Presence of precipitating factor	10 points
Diagnosis: Needs BWPS score of 45 or more to diagnose thyroid storm. *Score of 25 to 45 may indicate impending thyroid storm.* *Score less than 25 makes the diagnosis unlikely.*	

Table 3.
Burch–Wartofsky point scale (BWPS) scoring systems for thyroid storm.

Elevated T3/T4
Fever (38 °C/100.4 °F or greater)
Central nervous system (CNS) manifestation will be restlessness, delirium, psychosis/mental aberration, lethargy/somnolence, coma
Heart rate (130/min or higher)
Congestive heart failure (pulmonary edema to cardiogenic shock)
GI Manifestation (from vomiting to jaundice)

Table 4.
JTA scoring [7].

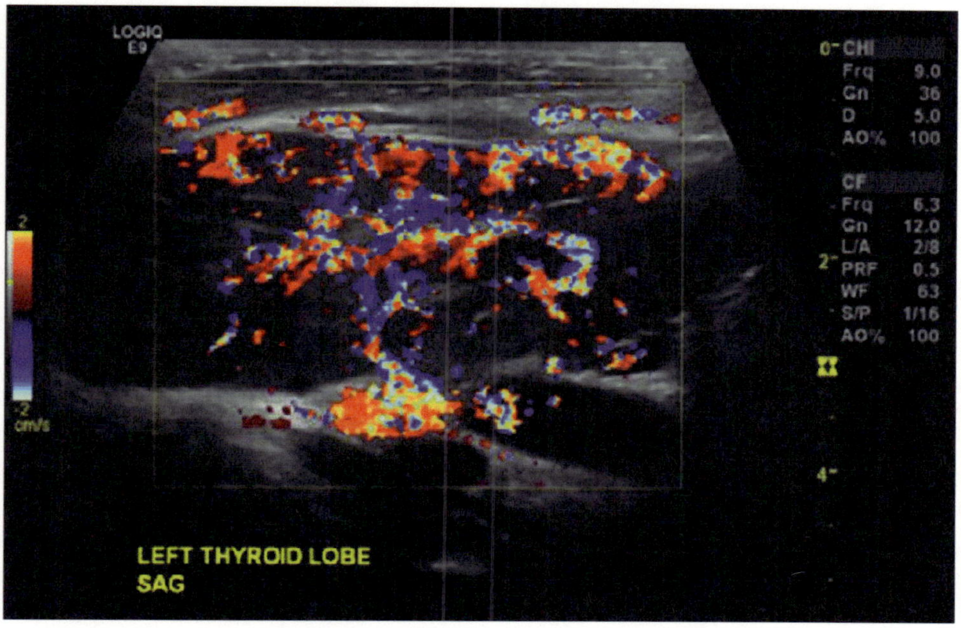

Figure 2.
POCUS showing hypervascular left lobe of thyroid gland.

symptoms along with fever, congestive heart failure (CHF), and tachycardia or combination of three features fever, GI/hepatic and congestive heart failure (CHF) or tachycardia. The JTA scoring system is more specific in diagnosis of thyroid storm.

Chest X-ray may show pulmonary congestion or pulmonary edema or cardiomegaly. ECG should be done which may reveal sinus tachycardia or tachyarrhythmia. Bedside POCUS may reveal a hypervascular thyroid gland (**Figure 2**). Patient may be breathless or short of breath and or hypotensive.

3.5 Management

One should not waste golden time in waiting for laboratory results, as thyroid storm is a medical emergency. Thyroid storm patients may present in shock, we should follow airway, breathing, circulation, deficit and exposer (ABCDE) approach and manage either cardiogenic or other dehydration causing hypovolemic shock in these patients. We should have continuous supportive management with advanced hemodynamic monitoring with intravenous fluids, core body temperature management, if required vasopressor and inotropes. These patients may have tachyarrhythmias and should be managed as per acute life support (ALS) protocol. These patients with thyroid storm need intensive care therapy unit admission and management.

The specific management strategies of thyroid storm are described in the following points.

1. Beta-blockers to control increased adrenergic tones.

2. Thioamide to reduce thyroid hormone synthesis.

3. Iodine solutions to reduce the release of thyroid hormones.

4. Glucocorticoid, PTU, and propranolol to reduce or block peripheral conversion of T4 to T3.

5. Bile acid sequestrant to reduce the enterohepatic recycling of thyroid hormones.

After ABCDE of supportive care, a beta-blocker should be started. Usually, propranolol 40–80 mg every 4 to 6 hours is administered.

PTU loading dose up to 1000 mg and followed by 250 mg every 4 hours or methimazole can be administered. PTU is preferred as it also has additional action of blocking peripheral conversion of T4 to T3. After 1 hour of PTU administration, 5 drops of supersaturated potassium iodide (SSKI) should be given per oral and repeat 6 hourly. This will prevent increase in synthesis of thyroid hormone due to iodine administration [9]. Hydrocortisone or dexamethasone, 100 mg intravenously and 2 mg Q 6 hourly respectively should also start. Cholestyramine 4 grams, 3 to 4 times will prevent enterohepatic recycling of thyroid hormones. Aspirin increases thyroid hormone levels and should be avoided in thyroid storm in these patients.

PTU decreases T3 by 45% in initial 24 hours of treatment. The methimazole causes more rapid normalization of T3 after weeks of treatment. Hence after initial stabilization, PTU should be changed to methimazole, if patient cannot take these medications orally can be given, and liquid preparation of the medications can be administered rectally. Patients with Graves' disease should be pretreated with beta-blocker, iodine therapy, and antithyroid medication before undergoing surgical intervention.

These medications are contraindicated due to allergy, thyroidectomy is required after treatment with Beta-blocker, steroids, cholestyramine, and iodine administration. The plasmapheresis should be the last resort if above measures fail [10].

4. Morbidity and mortality

Thyroid storm is fatal if not treated, usually heart failure, arrhythmias, or multiorgan failure leads to the death. If treatment starts, patients improve within 24 hours. The advanced age, neurological dysfunction upon admission, failure or delayed use of antithyroid medications or beta-blockers, requiring dialysis or mechanical ventilator increases the risk of death with poor prognosis [11].

5. Conclusion

Thyroid storm is an endocrine medical emergency, requiring early diagnosis and earlier management. Frequent precipitated by stress or acute illness or improper treatment of hyperthyroidism.

Thyroid storm or increased level of thyroxine or thyroid hormones causes multiple organ dysfunction or failure. Commonly manifested as fever, GI, central nervousness and cardiac dysfunctions, and arrhythmias. Thyroid storm diagnosed by clinical presentation, high index of suspicious, and use of scoring system. These patients can present in shock. Management should be supportive care, use of antithyroid medications, management of shock, antiarrhythmic therapy, and temperature management. Advanced age, neurological dysfunction at presentations, requirement of dialysis, invasive ventilation, and delay in antithyroid therapy will indicate a poor prognosis in thyroid storm.

Author details

Mohammad Zubair, Wael Khalaf, Zia Awan, Hossam Algallie, Nissar Shaikh and Gamal Al-Ameri*
Surgical Intensive Care, Hamad Medical Corporation, Doha, Qatar

*Address all correspondence to: drgamalabdulrahman@gmail.com

References

[1] Sarlis NJ, Gourgiolis L. Thyroid emergencies. Reviews in Endocrine & Metabolic Disorders. 2003;**4**:129

[2] Galindo RJ, Hurtado CR, Pasquel FJ, Garcia Tom R, et al. National trends in incidence, mortality and clinical outcomes of patients hospitalized for thyrotoxicosis with and without thyroid storm in United States 2004-13. Thyroid. 2019;**29**(1):36-43

[3] Akamizu T, Satoh T, Isozaki o et al. Japan thyroid association. Diagnostic, clinical features and incidence of thyroid storm based on national survey. Thyroid. 2012;**22**(7): 661-679

[4] Raza MA, Jain A, Mumtaz M, Mehmood T. Thyroid storm in a patient on chronic amiodarone treatment. Cureus. 2022;**14**(4):e24164

[5] De Ridder M, Sermeus AB, Urbain D, et al. Metastases to the thyroid gland, a report of six cases. European Journal of Internal Medicine. 2003;**14**(6):377-379

[6] Angell TE, Lechner MG, Nguyen CT, et al. Clinical features of hospital outcomes in thyroid storm; a retrospective cohort study. The Journal of Clinical Endocrinology and Metabolism. 2015;**100**(2):451-459

[7] Satoh T, Isozaki O, Suzuki A, Wakino S, Iburi T, Tsuboi K, et al. The Japanese thyroid association (JTA) score include elevated FT3/FT4 and presence of various clinical signs and symptoms. 2016 guidelines for the management of thyroid storm from the Japan thyroid association and Japan Endocrine Society (first edition). Endocrine Journal. 2016;**63**(12):1025-1064

[8] Bahn RS, Burch HB, Cooper DS, Garber JR, Greenlee MC, Klein I, et al. Hyperthyroidism and other causes of thyrotoxicosis: Management guidelines of the American Thyroid Association and American Association of Clinical Endocrinologists. Thyroid. 2011;**17**(3):456-520

[9] Jacobi J. Management of endocrine emergencies in intensive care unit. Journal of Pharmacy Practice. 2019;**322**(3):314-326

[10] Ba JH, Bq W, Wang YH, Shi YF. Therapeutic plasma exchange and continuous renal replacement therapy for severe hyperthyroidism and multi organs failure: A case report. World Journal of Clinical Cases. 2019;**7**(4):500-507

[11] Angel TE, Lechner MG, Nguyen CT, et al. Clinical features and hospital outcome in thyroid storm: A retrospective cohort study. The Journal of Clinical Endocrinology and Metabolism. 2015;**100**(2):451-459

Chapter 4

Diagnostics of Central and Autonomic Nervous System Dysfunction in Patients with Sepsis-Associated Encephalopathy

Irina Alexandrovna Savvina, Daria V. Ryzhkova, Kristina M. Bykova, Konstantin E. Lebedev, Anna Olegovna Petrova, Natalya V. Dryagina, Elena G. Potemkina and Eleonora T. Nazaralieva

Abstract

This chapter is devoted to monitoring of central and autonomic nervous system (ANS) in patients with verified sepsis to recognize the specific functional and anatomic changes in the brain and its important autonomic centers which is named sepsis-associated encephalopathy (SAE). Fluctuation of conscience level from agitation to delirium and coma, muscle tone, and severity of pain syndrome is evaluated with different scales (SOFA, SAPS II, RASS, CAM-ICU, FOUR, PBSS, BPS, MRC, MAS, CNS). Multimodal neuromonitoring includes EEG, EPs, ENMG, cerebral oxymetry, saturation in the bulb of the jugular vein, TCD, and neuroimaging (MRI, PET). Dysfunction of autonomic brainstem structures is detected with variational cardiointervalometry, pupillometry, thermometry (peripheral and central), photoplethysmography assessment of perfusion index, quantitative assessment of muscle strength on the MRC scale and MAS, and diagnostics of the severity of the PSH syndrome. Monitoring data help clinicians to make decisions on SAE patient management tactics.

Keywords: sepsis-associated encephalopathy, sepsis, neurophysiological monitoring, neuroimaging, multimodal assessment of neurological status, autonomic nervous system dysfunction

1. Introduction

The dysfunction of the central nervous system due to sepsis is realized in the form of sepsis-associated encephalopathy (SAE) with different levels of neurological deficit. SAE is an early manifestation of an infection of the body and may appear before other systemic signs of sepsis become apparent. SAE occurs in 70% of septic patients in critical condition and is associated with a higher mortality rate, longer hospital stay, poorer quality of life, and lower cognitive function scores than in other patients with sepsis without septic encephalopathy [1–3]. SAE can act as an independent predictor of mortality in severe sepsis and septic shock. The degree of its severity corresponds to the severity of the septic process [4].

The use of SOFA and SAPS II evaluation scales allows for determining the severity of the patient's condition for further solving therapeutic, prognostic, and legal issues. These scales are a clinical tool for assessing the patients' condition to predict the likelihood of developing a particular outcome, including death, disability, or long-term neurocognitive consequences. SAPS II was found to be more accurate than APACHE II, a similar intensive care classification score, and is commonly used in studies to compare morbidity and outcomes among patients.

2. Diagnostics of central nervous system dysfunction in patients with SAE

Patients with verified sepsis according to the international consensus definitions of sepsis and septic shock sepsis-3 (Third International Consensus Definitions for Sepsis and Septic Shock, 2016), undergo clinical, laboratorial, radiological, and functional examination in order to identify nonspecific and specific functional and structural changes in the central nervous system inherent in acute cerebral injury, caused by a systemic infection. According to a number of authors, the absence of specific markers for the diagnosis of SAE complicates the diagnosis [4–6].

2.1 Neurological assessment

Impaired consciousness is revealed in a significant proportion of patients with sepsis, and it may even precede the manifestations of the underlying disease. At the same time, the presence of signs of a disorder of consciousness sharply worsens the prognosis. There are various clinical variants of the course of SAE from acute minimal changes in mental status and behavioral disorders (inattention, disorientation, and excitement) to delirium and coma [7]. Delirium is defined as a single syndrome in which a number of different etiological causes cause a relatively consistent pattern of acute generalized cognitive disorders [8].

A patient with sepsis and SAE is given a comprehensive diagnosis of disorders of the level of consciousness, in the case of coma—brainstem reflexes to assess the depth of coma, in the case of fluctuations in the level of consciousness—agitation, excitement, aggression, and confusion to a hypo-active state, for objective dynamic monitoring of a life-threatening condition, timely decision-making for therapeutic tactics for delirium relief, transfer of the patient to a state of medically induced coma (neurovegetative stabilization), and respiratory support. Dynamic behavioral assessment of the severity of pain syndrome in a patient with SAE gives clinicians a tool for choosing the regimen and doses of analgesic drugs from NSAIDs and paracetamol to opioids in the structure of neurovegetative blockade.

Assessment of muscle tone is extremely important due to the rapid development of critical condition polyneuromyopathy in patients with sepsis, which undoubtedly affects the rehabilitation potential of a septic patient when the condition is stabilized. We consider it appropriate and recommend using the following scales for patients with sepsis and SAE to assess the dysfunction of the central and autonomous parts of the nervous system:

- RASS (Richmond Agitation-Sedation Scale)—description of the degree of aggression of the patient or the level of sedation depth;

- CAM-ICU Scale (Confusion Assessment Method-Intensive Care Unit)—assessment of confusion (**Appendix**, **Figure** 7); assessment of hypo-active, hyperactive, or mixed form of delirium;

- Coma Scale FOUR (Full Outline of UnResponsiveness)—more precisely details the neurological status, recognizes the locked-in syndrome, evaluates brainstem reflexes, evaluates the respiratory pattern, and identifies various stages of brain dislocation. FOUR score is a new coma scale that was recently developed and validated in adults as a proposed replacement for the Glasgow Coma Scale (GCS) and it is not reliant on verbal response;

- PBSS (Pittsburg BrainStem Score)—used to assess brainstem reflexes in patients in a coma and to assess the depth of coma of nontraumatic genesis;

- BPS (Behavioral Pain Scale)—objectification of pain syndrome;

- MRC scale (Medical Research Council Weakness Scale)—quantitative assessment of muscle strength; used in awake patients in consciousness;

- MAS (Modified Ashworth Scale)—assessment of spasticity; used in patients with increased muscle tone of the extremities due to cerebral damage;

- CNS (Canadian Neurological Scale)—rapid assessment of the level of neurological deficit associated with acute cerebrovascular events.

Surviving patients are often left with long-term cognitive impairments that can lead to disability. There is increasing evidence that SAE can cause long-term cognitive impairment, including changes in the speed of mental processing, decreased memory, attention, and visual–spatial abilities [9]. They can persist for several years after the diagnosis of SAE, affecting functional abilities, quality of life, and the ability to return to work. Depending on the degree of disorders (e.g., mild, moderate, or severe), the presence of this disease can be a great burden for both family members and caregivers. Many patients diagnosed with SAE have chronic neurocognitive effects for 6 years after discharge from the intensive care unit [10]. A small series of cases showed that several months after discharge from the intensive care unit, all patients had severe memory and attention disorders [11]. These restrictions arose when performing basic everyday tasks, such as eating, bathing, and various household activities. Other important neuropsychiatric diseases that are present in surviving patients are depression and anxiety. The prevalence and severity of these mental disorders in patients vary from 10–58% [12].

2.2 Laboratory diagnostic markers

With the development of SAE from the standpoint of pathophysiology, the endothelium and blood–brain barrier (BBB) are damaged, resulting in the destruction of proteins with their subsequent release into the bloodstream. These peptides can be considered as markers of BBB integrity. In the study by Barichello et al., plasma levels of occludin, claudin-5, zonula occludens-1 (ZO-1), procalcitonin, and lactate were evaluated in patients with sepsis [13]. Occludin and ZO-1 were elevated and positively correlated with the severity of the disease. The prognostic value of the ZO-1 level for in-hospital mortality was comparable to the lactate level [14].

In another study, Wang et al., the diameter of the optic nerve sheath (ONSD) was measured using ultrasound in rabbits with SAE and the levels of neurospecific enolase (NSE), astroglial protein S100B, tumor necrosis factor-α (TNF-α) were determined by enzyme immunoassay. According to the results of the study, changes in ONSD (increased over time) correlated with NSE and S100B. ONSD monitoring has shown a high prognostic value in SAE [14].

It is known that S100B and NSE are biomarkers of brain damage in traumatic brain injury, cerebral stroke, and hypoxic–ischemic encephalopathy. A retrospective analysis of a sepsis cohort reported that an NSE concentration > 12.5 μg/L was independently associated with 23% and 29% increased risk of 30-day mortality and delirium, respectively [15]. In the studies of Yao et al., the clinical significance of S100B and NSE in blood serum for the diagnosis of SAE and evaluation of its prognosis was studied. Studies have shown that serum concentrations of S100B in patients with SAE were significantly higher than in patients without SAE. The efficacy and sensitivity of serum S100B in the diagnosis of SAE were high, but they had low specificity. Compared with NSE, serum S100B was better suited both for the diagnosis of SAE and predicting the outcome of sepsis [16]. Also, in a study by Piazza et al., it was shown that the level of S100B protein in patients with SAE was elevated but did not correlate with the Glasgow Coma scale (GCS) at admission, the electroencephalogram pattern (EEG) or the SOFA scale score. It follows from the above that in sepsis, an increase in S100B does not allow physicians to predict neurological recovery [17].

The prognostic value of light (NfL) and heavy (NfH) neurofilament chain levels as biomarkers of neuroaxonal injury in patients with sepsis-associated encephalopathy were measured by Ehler J. et al. in the prospective, pilot observational study (2019) [18]. According to the results of researchers, the plasma and CSF NfL levels were higher in patients with SAE and correlated with the severity of SAE and a poor functional outcome. As the result, there was found a correlation between the higher value of CSF NfL levels and mortality.

2.3 Neuroimaging

2.3.1 Magnetic resonance imaging

Neuroimaging in patients with SAE gives different results. In some patients, the results of magnetic resonance imaging (MRI) of the brain reflect the normal state of the cortical–subcortical structures and the brainstem, in other patients, acute damage is observed. In the case of acute injury, MRI reveals, in particular, multiple ischemic strokes or white matter lesions in the semi-oval center (mainly at the level of Virchow-Robin spaces). MRI signs of septic acute cerebral injury are presented in **Figure 1.**

According to Sharshar et al., the severity of damage in the central nervous system is associated with the severity of sepsis and inversely correlates with the scores on the GCS [19]. A lesion in the white matter of the brain corresponds to vasogenic edema (e.g., an increased signal on a T2-weighted image and a reduced signal on a diffusion-weighted image). Data published by Piazza et al., indicate that the size and number of foci of brain damage vary significantly among patients with SAE [20].

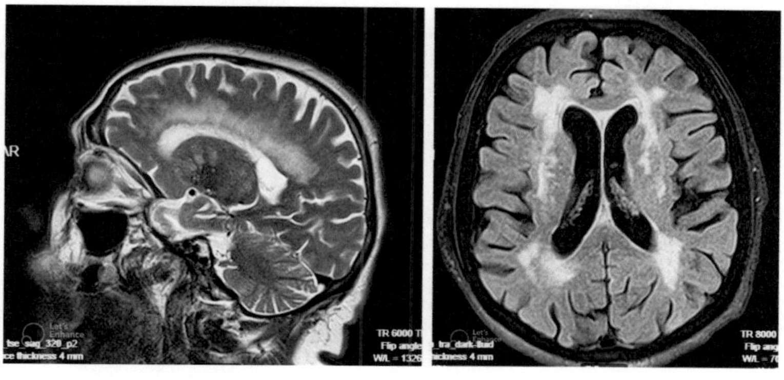

Figure 1.
A, B. MRI of the brain of patient P., 75 y.o., on the 5th day of diagnostics of SAE. T2- WI (A), flair pulse sequence (B). In the subcortical, periventricular parts of the white matter of the brain, multiple different-sized foci of hyperintense signal are visualized, ranging in size from 3 to 14 mm, with a tendency to merge, in places of a draining nature, probably of a dyscirculatory genesis. Pronounced zones of leukoaraiosis are noted periventricularly to both horns of the lateral ventricles. Rating on the scale RASS +2 points; CAM-ICU—Delirium is present.

Posterior reversible encephalopathy syndrome (PRES) is a clinical radiological syndrome characterized by headache, confusion, seizures, and visual impairment [21], which is associated with edema of the white matter, primarily affecting the posterior regions—the occipital and parietal lobes to varying degrees is often diagnosed with sepsis. According to Fugate, who published the results of a Mayo Clinic study, PRES was associated with sepsis in 7–24% of patients [22].

2.3.2 Positron emission tomography

Metabolic changes detected in brain structures according to positron emission tomography with 18F-fluorodeoxyglucose (18F-FDG PET) in patients with SAE at different stages of the course of sepsis, hypometabolism of various parts of the cerebral cortex are concerned.

Figures 2–4 show the PET data of the patients with SAE on the 5th, 6th' and 28th days from the diagnosis of sepsis, SAE. The 18F-FDG PET images revealed signs of diffuse hypometabolism in the cerebral cortex, which may reflect not only structural lesions but also functional ones.

However, it should be taken into account that patients with acute cerebral damage of different severity due to sepsis are often transported for imaging and receive hypnotic agents in the structure of intensive therapy, in particular, propofol, which causes nonspecific changes in metabolism in the cerebral cortex to a lesser extent than other hypnotics and anesthetics (e.g., thiopental sodium).

Thus, neuroimaging in patients with SAE gives different results—from the absence of pathological changes to acute cerebral damage, including vasogenic edema of white matter in the periventricular parts of both hemispheres, a pattern of hypoperfusion of the cerebral cortex, and hypometabolism in various parts of the cerebral cortex.

2.4 Transcranial doppler

Cerebral perfusion pressure (CPP) under condition of violated cerebrovascular autoregulation can lead to global cerebral ischemia (low CPP), and hemorrhage and

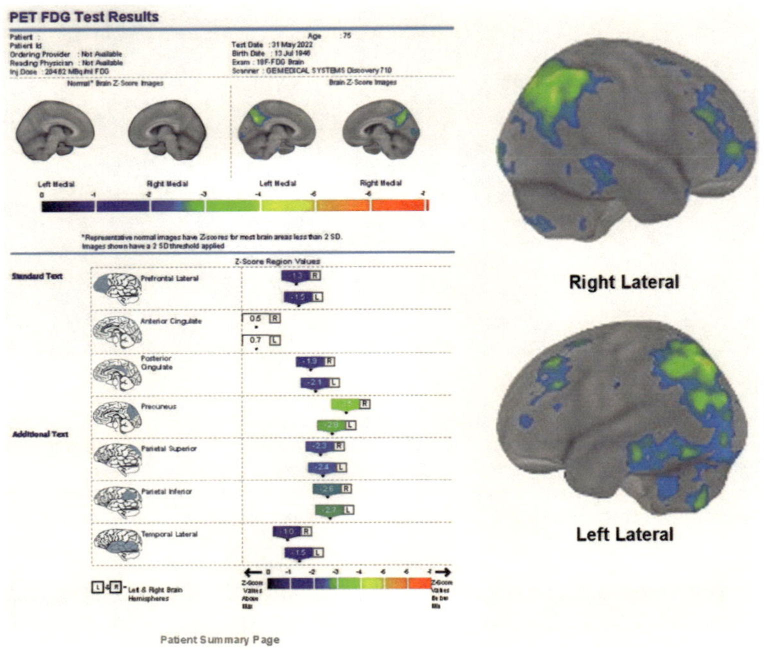

Figure 2.
18F-FDG PET of the brain on the 5th day after SAE diagnostics in patient P., 75 years old. PET was performed under sedation with propofol 2 mg/kg/h. Glucose hypometabolism in the cerebral cortex in different areas (marked in green). A decrease in glucose metabolism in the parietal lobes. Score according to RASS is a + 2 points, and in CAM-ICU—Delirium is present.

brain edema (high CPP). Both events may cause neuronal damage and sepsis-associated delirium (SAD). Pfister et al. introduced that in 16 patients impaired autoregulation 48 hours after the onset of sepsis was found, and SAD was diagnosed [23].

The transcranial doppler (TCD)—derived index of autoregulation Mx is used for the assessment of the status of autoregulation; this index has been already calculated for many different clinical conditions: in traumatic brain injury, carotid artery diseases, vasospasm, volunteers, and in sepsis [23, 24].

In the study, Schramm et al. show that autoregulation is impaired in the majority of patients with severe sepsis and septic shock during the first 2 days [25]. Daily measurement of index Mx in patients with verified sepsis during the first 4 days found increased index Mx in the first 2 days, and, thus, impairment of autoregulation which was associated with the occurrence of SAD, suggesting that autoregulation is one of the factors contributing to SAD.

The association between severe sepsis and septic shock and increased cerebral vascular resistance as assessed by TCD estimated pulsatility index (PI) and resistance index (RI) was previously reported (PI = systolic velocity—(diastolic velocity/mean velocity); RI = systolic velocity—(diastolic velocity/systolic velocity)) [26]. The study of Algebaly et al., showed that pediatric septic patients with SAE had significantly higher PI and RI than their counterparts without SAE [27].

Another study on septic patients by Pierrakos et al., identified TCD-derived PI in the first post-admission day as a significant predictor of subsequent SAE with good sensitivity and specificity [28]. Moreover, the study of Crippa et al., which recruited 100 patients with sepsis, reported a significant association between sepsis-associated brain dysfunction and altered cerebral autoregulation detected by TCD [29].

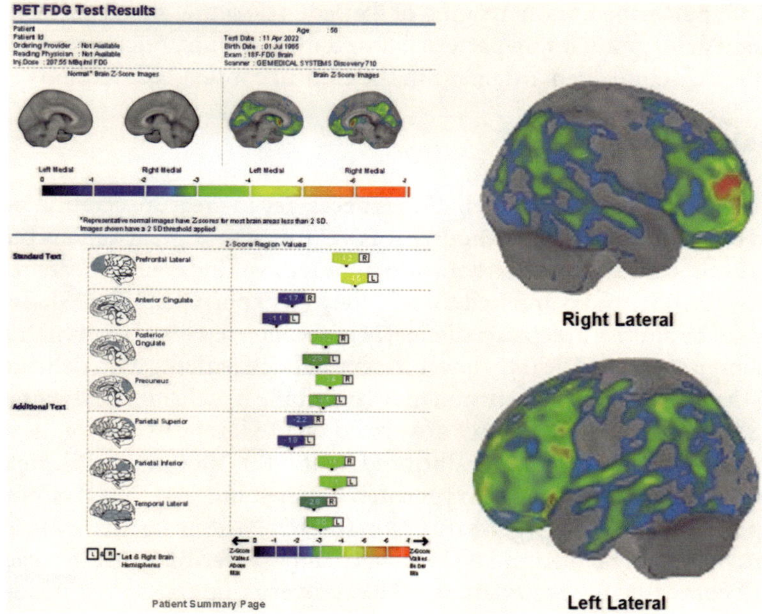

Figure 3.
18F-FDG PET of the brain in 6 days after SAE diagnostics in patient S., 56 years old. Glucose hypometabolism in various parts of the cerebral cortex (marked in green). The study was performed without sedation. The score according to FOUR scale is 6 points; to PBSS is 10 points; and to CNS is 3,5 points.

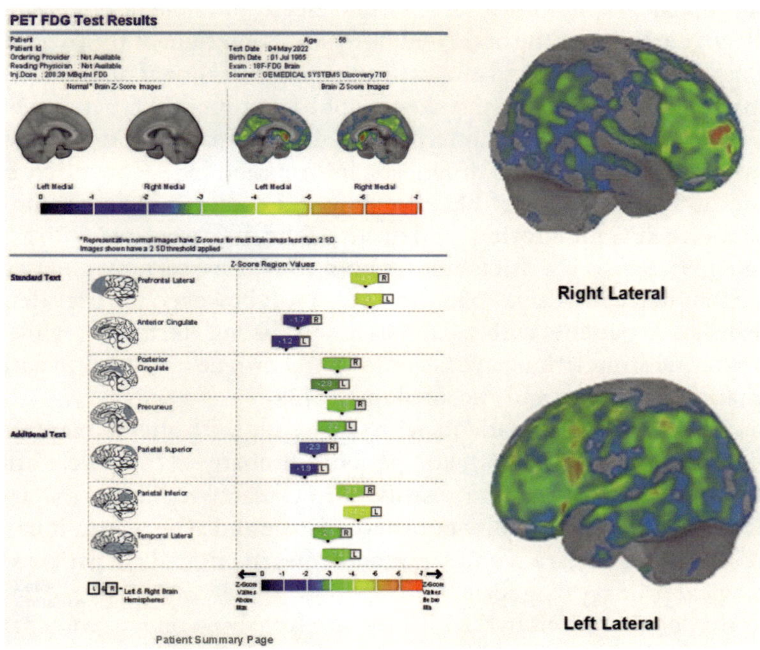

Figure 4.
18F-FDG PET of the brain on the 28th day of sepsis and SAE in patient S., 56 years old. Glucose hypometabolism persists in various parts of the cerebral cortex (marked in green). The study was performed on the background of sedation with propofol. The score according to GCS is 13 points; to FOUR scale is 10 points; to PBSS is 11 points; and to CNS is 4,5 points before sedation starts.

Sanz et al., performed brain imaging of 49 pediatric septic shock patients, and the most frequent acute brain lesion patterns, found on neuroimaging, were ischemia and cerebritis (i.e., cerebral edema/damage in the clinical context of infection) [30].

2.5 Cerebral oxymetry

Determination of cerebral oxygenation is necessary to measure cerebral perfusion. It is carried out with following methods: invasive (direct)—jugular venous bulb oxygen saturation, brain tissue oxygen tension, and noninvasive (indirect)—near-infrared spectroscopy (NIRS), and computed tomography (CT) perfusion [31–33]. Cerebral perfusion may be altered in sepsis patients [24]. Recently, cerebral oxygenation has also been shown to be significantly lower in septic shock patients with delirium [34], suggesting that poor cerebral perfusion may contribute to delirium development.

In NIRS, a sensor and light source are placed on the forehead, where they emit and receive varying wavelengths of near-infrared light (700–1000 nm) [35], representing changes in oxygenated- and deoxygenated hemoglobin [36]. NIRS noninvasively measures peripheral tissue oxygen saturation (StO2). NIRS measurements for the StO2 initial, StO2 occlusion, and StO2 recovery slope were abnormal in patients with septic shock compared to sepsis patients. The recovery slope was most strongly associated with organ dysfunction and mortality [37].

2.6 Neurophysiological monitoring

2.6.1 Electroencephalography

Electroencephalography (EEG) allows rapid electrophysiological measurements of the bioelectric activity of the brain and its dysfunction right at the patient's bedside and complements the clinical and neuroimaging assessment of patients with encephalopathy. Both the progressive slowing of background EEG activity with an increase in cerebral insufficiency and a decrease in EEG reactivity to external stimuli provide important diagnostic and prognostic information [38]. Convulsive seizures and periodic discharges (a type of EEG anomaly) are common in patients in critical condition, require EEG monitoring for detection, and are associated with an unfavorable outcome [39]. Sepsis is a risk factor for both convulsive seizures and periodic discharges, including convulsive epileptic status [40]; however, the prevalence of all these disorders in patients with sepsis has not yet been determined, while EEG changes to external stimulation have become a good prognostic factor in patients with acute traumatic brain injury and encephalopathy [38].

In a prospective analysis of patients with sepsis, and with altered mental status, seizures without convulsions (11%), and periodic discharges (25%) were often detected. It was also proved that the absence of EEG reactivity in the first days of sepsis was associated with mortality both at discharge and after 1 year. It has been shown that EEG reactivity is a predictor of outcomes in critically ill patients with a non-neurological primary diagnosis.

A wide range of alterations in the EEG pattern have been registered in patients with sepsis and SAE: progressive slowing of the normal alpha rhythm, appearance of theta to delta activity, triphasic waves, and malignant burst suppression in severe malignant encephalopathy [5, 41, 42]. According to Young et al., EEG patterns have been classified into four categories of increasing severity of SAE [43]. Examples of EEG changes according to the stage of SAE are demonstrated in **Figures 5** and **6**.

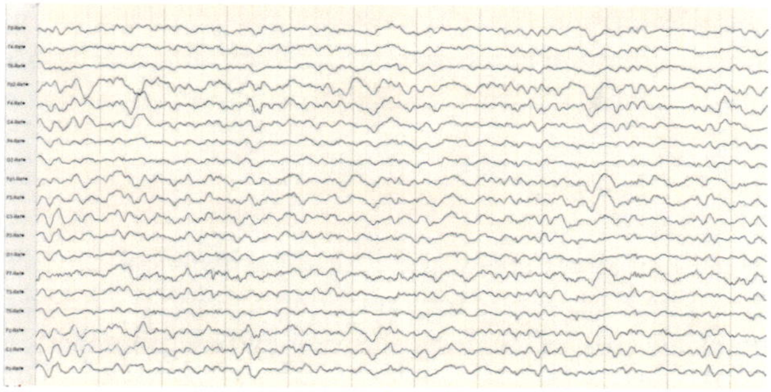

Figure 5.
EEG of patient S., 56 years old, in 6 and 16 days after SAE diagnostics, coma 1. EEG— Electroencephalography. Slow-wave activity dominates. The record is represented by the polymorphic activity of the predominantly theta range. There is an interhemispheric asymmetry: in the left hemisphere, the amplitude of biopotentials is reduced (20 mv); in the right hemisphere, mainly in the frontal-temporal leads, groups of delta waves of increased amplitude (70 mv) in combination with acute waves are recorded. EEG data indicate gross widespread changes with a focus on pathological activity in the frontotemporal region of the right hemisphere.

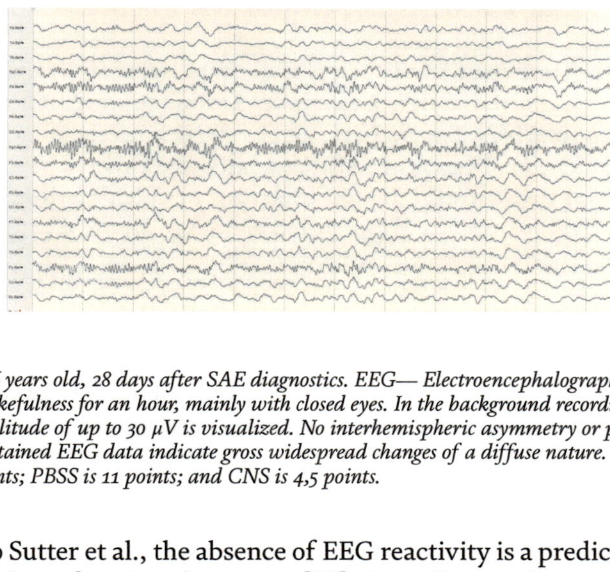

Figure 6.
EEG of patient S., 56 years old, 28 days after SAE diagnostics. EEG— Electroencephalography. Registration in a state of relaxed wakefulness for an hour, mainly with closed eyes. In the background recording, polymorphic activity with an amplitude of up to 30 μV is visualized. No interhemispheric asymmetry or paroxysmal activity was recorded. The obtained EEG data indicate gross widespread changes of a diffuse nature. The score according to FOUR scale is 10 points; PBSS is 11 points; and CNS is 4,5 points.

According to Sutter et al., the absence of EEG reactivity is a predictor of mortality but does not predict a functional outcome [38]. According to the concept of Moruzzi G., the reactivity of the EEG to external simulation depends on the preservation of brain stem structures, such as the ascending reticular formation, but the reactivity of the EEG does not necessarily reflect higher brain activity [44]. The results of fundamental research by Moruzzi et al., emphasize the importance of secondary brain dysfunction and, perhaps, precisely brain stem dysfunction in critical conditions. The researchers also found that the sedative effect was associated with a decrease in nonconvulsive seizures or periodic discharges and a lack of EEG reactivity. It is possible that the sedative effect interferes with the reactivity test during the EEG. Nevertheless, as noted in a study by Shehabi et al., continuous sedation is associated with increased mortality [45].

EEG monitoring gives us an excellent opportunity to improve the ability to predict and prevent seizures, predict and potentially prevent neuronal disorders [39].

The diagnosis of SAE may precede neurological changes in patients who underwent EEG monitoring [46]. In two-thirds of the cases, violations on the EEG did not give any clinical manifestations. Nevertheless, the progressive slowing of background EEG activity with an increase in cerebral insufficiency, and a decrease in EEG reactivity to external stimuli, provide important diagnostic and prognostic information.

2.6.2 Evoked potentials

The functional state of the sensory and motor pathways of the brainstem in patients with SAE can be assessed by registering multimodal evoked potentials (EPs): motor-evoked potentials (MEPs), somatosensory-evoked potentials (SSEPs), visual-avoked potentials (VAPs), and brainstem auditory-evoked potentials (BAEPs).

EPs measure brain responses to sensory stimulation [47], including responses generated by subcortical structures (BAEPs, SSERs), thalamocortical input to the primary sensory cortices, and intrinsic cortical activity [48]. Abnormal EPs are present in the majority of septic patients [41]. The clinical examination may be less sensitive than electrophysiological methods in the diagnosis of SAE. Rinaldi et al., studied the changes in A-line autoregression index (AAI) induced by postsurgical sepsis [49]. It was shown that the occurrence of sepsis significantly reduces AAI. Thus, the measurement of AAI has the potential to be a reliable diagnostic test to identify subclinical SAE [49].

Alteration in the latency or amplitude of the somatosensory-evoked potentials has been frequently reported in this patient population [50], and it is not influenced by sedative medications [42]. Subcortical (i.e., N20–N23 interlatency) and cortical (N20–N70 interlatency) pathways of SSEPs are impaired early in 34% and 84% of 68 septic patients [51]. EPs are useful for assessing SAE in sedated critically ill patients as in contrast to EEG, their latencies are slightly altered by sedatives [42].

3. Functional assessment of ANS in patients with SAE

Assessment of the functional state of ANS is carried out by calculating the autonomic Kerdo index, assessing the severity of pain syndrome using BPS; BrainStem Scores (FOUR, PBSS); trends in the hemodynamic profile of a patient with invasive measurement of systemic hemodynamics, assessment of HRV (variational cardiointervalography), thermometry (peripheral and central), photoplethysmography assessment of perfusion index, quantitative assessment of muscle strength on the MRC scale and MAS; diagnostics the severity of the PSH syndrome in the case of its development with gross dysfunction of the oral parts of the brainstem [52].

3.1 Pupillometry

In recent years, a quantitative evaluation of the pupillary light reflex (PLR) using portable pupillometers has become available in the ICU [53, 54].

Pupillary size is controlled by the balance between sympathetic and parasympathetic systems, integrated at the midbrain level, as well as by neuronal activity of the locus coeruleus, colliculi, and cingulate cortex. It is known that the cholinergic parasympathetic pathways of the brain play the important role in the recognition of infection and integrative response to systemic infection [55].

Various neurotransmitter systems are involved in the control of cortical activity, which may also affect pupillary size, in particular acetylcholine and norepinephrine [55].

Several researchers have supposed that quantitative PLR (expressed as the percentage pupillary constriction to a calibrated light stimulus) may improve the prediction of neurological outcomes after cardiac arrest [56, 57].

Quantitative pupillometry is used for the assessment of pupillary function, in particular, the neurological pupil index (NPi). The NPi is a scalar value (between 0 and 5) that is calculated based on an algorithm that accounts for several measured pupillary variables, including size, percentage constriction, constriction velocity, dilation velocity, and latency [58]. The NPi is only minimally influenced by medications, in particular, opioids and ambient light, and it accounts for individual baseline pupil size [58, 59]. This is especially valuable due to the fact that patients with SAE in a coma require a therapeutic technique—neurovegetative blockade, implying the use of opioids, hypnotics, and a2-adrenoagonists.

The diagnostic value of the method for monitoring the function of the brainstem for making clinical decisions—withdrawal to the diagnostic window, cessation of neurovegetative blockade—is very high. Since the method is increasingly being used to predict outcomes after cardiac arrest [60], we believe that a dynamic assessment of the diameter and reactivity of the pupil—the most important autonomous PLR—using the automated infrared pupillometry method will allow monitoring the functional state of the brainstem (midbrain) and identify the earliest changes in sepsis in the central nervous system. In one study, scientists observed only a weak correlation between NPI (i.e., one pupillometry-derived variable) and the Mxa, which is an index assessing cerebral AR. This correlation remained significant in the septic patients' group, while no correlation was observed in non-septic patients [61].

3.2 Electroneuromyography

Qualitative electromyography (EMG) reveals myopathic changes in the study of muscles: a decrease in the amplitude and a shortening of the duration of the action potential [62]. One study assessed the frequency and time of onset of neuromuscular disorders using electromyography in patients with systemic inflammatory response syndrome (SIRS) and/or sepsis [63]. Electromyography and conduction velocity measurements were performed on days 2–5 after admission to the intensive care unit. In patients, electromyography revealed signs of neuromuscular abnormality. The means of compound muscle action potential amplitudes of the median and ulnar nerves were decreased.

Special electrophysiological examination—nerve conduction studies (NCS) and EMG are used in critically ill patients from time to time because of the intensity of work in ICUs—heavy patient workload and high cost [64]. Usually, NCS registrate reduced compound muscle action potentials; in the case of (coexistent) critical illness polyneuropathy, reduced sensory nerve action potentials, and normal or slightly reduced nerve conduction velocity [65]. According to Stevens et al., EMG examination of patients in ICU with sepsis revealed primary distal axonal nerve degeneration involving both sensory and motor fibers without signs of demyelination or inflammation [66].

4. Conclusion

Despite significant advances in the treatment of sepsis, SAE is still associated with the development of acute cerebral insufficiency, severe autonomic dysfunction in the form of autonomic distress syndrome and high mortality due to dystrophic and necrobiotic changes in the autonomic nuclei of the ANS, as shown by studies of pathologists. The revealed changes prove that the septic process causes not only functionally reversible but also morphological pathological changes in the brain resulting from damage to structural and anatomical formations of the ANS, which can serve as an application point for the development of treatment methods for SAE.

The creation of a universal tool for assessing the severity of encephalopathy and determining the dynamics of the restoration of neurocognitive functions, in a particular patient will help the practitioner to evaluate the effectiveness of therapeutic measures, as well as complement specific neuroprotective or metabolotropic therapy. The sensitivity and specificity of each of the considered neuroimaging, neurophysiological research methods, and options for monitoring the functional state of the central and ANS in sepsis will be determined—the next important step in research. Obviously, the development of an algorithm for diagnosing, predicting the course and outcome, and intensive therapy of patients with SAE is ahead. We are convinced that only a multidisciplinary approach for solving such complex tasks will allow us to see results in the coming years.

Conflict of interest

There is no conflict of interest.

Abbreviations

BPS	Behavioral Pain Scale
CAM-ICU	Confusion Assessment Method-Intensive Care Unit
CBF	cerebral blood flow
CNS	Canadian Neurological Scale
CSF	cerebro-spinal fluid
EEG	electroencephalogram
ENMG	electroneuromyography
Eps	evoked potentials
FOUR	Full Outline of UnResponsiveness Score
GCS	Glasgow Coma Scale
HRV	heart rate variability
ICU	Intensive Care Unit
MAS	Modified Ashworth Scale
MRC	Medical Research Council Weakness Scale
MRI	magnetic resonance imaging
ONSD	optic nerve sheath diameter
PBSS	Pittsburgh Brainstem Score
PET	positron emission tomography
PLR	pupillary light reflex
PSH	paroxysmal sympathetic hyperactivity syndrome
RASS	Richmond Agitation-Sedation Scale
SAD	sepsis-associated delirium
SAE	sepsis-associated encephalopathy

SAPS II	Simplified Acute Physiology Score
SOFA	Sequential Organ Failure Assessment score
T2-WI	T2-weighted image
TCD	transcranial Doppler

Appendix

Confusion assessment method for intensive care unit (CAM-ICU).

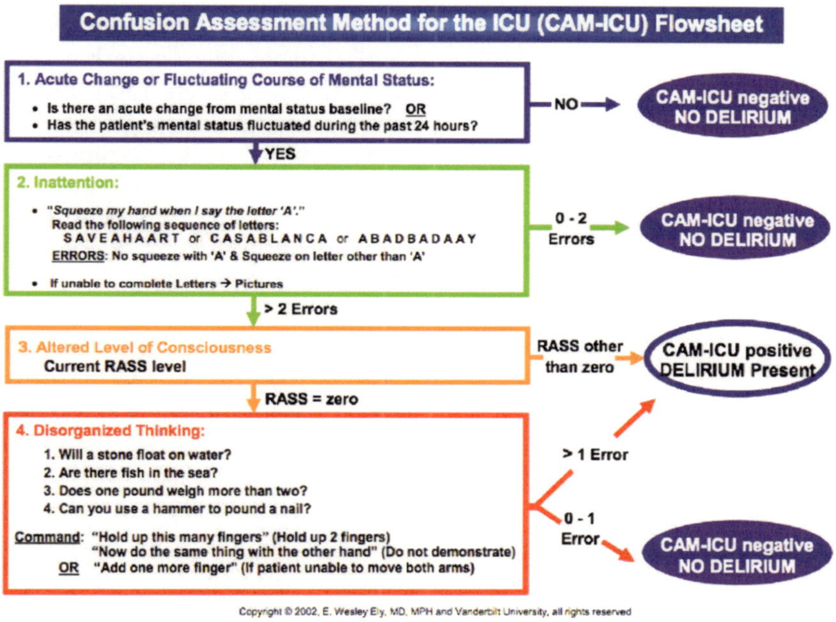

Figure 7.
Confusion assessment method for the ICU (CAM-ICU) flowsheet [67].

Author details

Irina Alexandrovna Savvina*, Daria V. Ryzhkova, Kristina M. Bykova, Konstantin E. Lebedev, Anna Olegovna Petrova, Natalya V. Dryagina, Elena G. Potemkina and Eleonora T. Nazaralieva
Almazov National Medical Research Center, Saint Petersburg, Russian Federation

*Address all correspondence to: irinasavvina@mail.ru

References

[1] Zhao L, Li Y, Wang Y, et al. Non-hepatic Hyperammonemia: A potential therapeutic target for Sepsis-associated encephalopathy. CNS & Neurological Disorders Drug Targets. 2021;**21**(9):738-751. DOI: 10.2174/1871527321666211221161534

[2] Gilmore EJ, Gaspard N, Choi HA, et al. Acute brain failure in severe sepsis: A prospective study in the medical intensive care unit utilizing continuous EEG monitoring. Intensive Care Medicine. 2015;**41**:686-694. DOI: 10.1007/s00134-015-3709-1

[3] Savvina IA, Zabrodskaya YM, Sebelev KI, Petrova AO, Bodareva NV. Septical encephalopathy: Pathophysiology, pathomorphology, clinical syndromes and therapeutic tactics. Neurosurgery and Pediatric Neurology. 2017;**4**(17):20-33

[4] Eggers V, Schilling A, Kox WJ, et al. Septic encephalopathy. Diagnosis und therapy. Anaesthesist. 2003;**52**:294-303. DOI: 10.1007/s00101-003-0496-9

[5] Gofton TE, Young GB. Sepsis-associated encephalopathy. Nature Reviews. Neurology. 2012;**8**:557-566. DOI: 10.1038/nrneurol.2012.183

[6] Della Giovampaola M, Cavalli I, Mascia L. Neuropsychological outcome of critically ill patients with severe infection. Biomedicine. 2022;**10**:526

[7] Fesenko OV, Sinopalnikov AI, Filatov VV, et al. Clinical aspects of septic encephalopathy. Clinical Medical Russian Journal. 2016;**94**:67-70. DOI: 10.18821/0023-2149-2016-94-1-67-70

[8] Sekhon S, Fischer MA, Marwaha R. Excited Delirium. Treasure Island, FL: StatPearls Publishing; 2022

[9] Lamar CD, Hurley RA, Taber KH. Sepsis-associated encephalopathy: Review of the neuropsychiatric manifestations and cognitive outcome. The Journal of Neuropsychiatry and Clinical Neurosciences. 2011;**23**:237-241. DOI: 10.1176/jnp.23.3.jnp237

[10] Rothenhäusler HB, Ehrentraut S, Stoll C, et al. The relationship between cognitive performance and employment and health status in long-term survivors of the acute respiratory distress syndrome: Results of an exploratory study. General Hospital Psychiatry. 2001;**23**:90-96. DOI: 10.1016/s0163-8343(01)00123-2

[11] Iwashyna TJ, Ely EW, Smith DM, et al. Long-term cognitive impairment and functional disability among survivors of severe sepsis. JAMA. 2010;**304**:1787-1794. DOI: 10.1001/jama.2010.1553

[12] Jackson JC, Mitchell N, Hopkins RO. Cognitive functioning, mental health, and quality of life in ICU survivors: An overview. Critical Care Clinics. 2009;**25**:615. DOI: 10.1016/j.ccc.2009.04.005

[13] Barichello T, Generoso JS, Singer M, et al. Biomarkers for sepsis: More than just fever and leukocytosis-a narrative review. Critical Care London English. 2022;**26**:14. DOI: 10.1186/s13054-021-03862-5

[14] Wang J, Yang M, Xu H, et al. Diagnostic value of ONSD in sepsis associated encephalopathy of New Zealand rabbits. Brain Research Bulletin. 2022;**179**:68-73. DOI: 10.1016/j.brainresbull.2021.12.002

[15] Anderson BJ, Reilly JP. Admission plasma levels of the neuronal injury

marker neuron-specific enolase are associated with mortality and delirium in sepsis. Journal of Critical Care. 2016;**36**:18-23

[16] Yao B, Zhang L-N, Ai Y-H, et al. Serum S100β is a better biomarker than neuron-specific enolase for sepsis-associated encephalopathy and determining its prognosis: A prospective and observational study. Neurochemical Research. 2014;**39**:1263-1269. DOI: 10.1007/s11064-014-1308-0

[17] Piazza O, Russo E, Cotena S, et al. Elevated S100B levels do not correlate with the severity of encephalopathy during sepsis. British Journal of Anaesthesia. 2007;**99**:518-521. DOI: 10.1093/bja/aem201

[18] Ehler J, Petzold A, Wittstock M, Kolbaske S, Gloger M, Henschel J, et al. The prognostic value of neurofilament levels in patients with sepsis-associated encephalopathy—A prospective, pilot observational study. PLoS One. 2019;**14**:e0211184

[19] Sharshar T, Carlier R, Bernard F, et al. Brain lesions in septic shock: A magnetic resonance imaging study. Intensive Care Medicine. 2007;**33**:798-806. DOI: 10.1007/s00134-007-0598-y

[20] Piazza O, Cotena S, De Robertis E, et al. Sepsis associated encephalopathy studied by MRI and cerebral spinal fluid S100B measurement. Neurochemical Research. 2009;**34**:1289-1292. DOI: 10.1007/s11064-008-9907-2

[21] Hinchey J, Chaves C, Appignani B, et al. A reversible posterior leukoencephalopathy syndrome. The New England Journal of Medicine. 1996;**334**:494-500. DOI: 10.1056/NEJM199602223340803

[22] Fugate JE, Claassen DO, Cloft HJ, et al. Posterior reversible encephalopathy syndrome: Associated clinical and radiologic findings. Mayo Clinic Proceedings. 2010;**85**:427-432. DOI: 10.4065/mcp.2009.0590

[23] Pfister D, Siegemund M, Dell-Kuster S, Smielewski P, Rüegg S, Strebel SP, et al. Cerebral perfusion in sepsis-associated delirium. Critical Care London. 2008;**12**(3):R63

[24] Steiner LA, Pfister D, Strebel SP, Radolovich D, Smielewski P, Czosnyka M. Near-infrared spectroscopy can monitor dynamic cerebral autoregulation in adults. Neurocritical Care. 2009;**10**(1):122-128

[25] Schramm P, Klein KU, Falkenberg L, Berres M, Closhen D, Werhahn KJ, et al. Impaired cerebrovascular autoregulation in patients with severe sepsis and sepsis-associated delirium. Critical Care. 2012;**16**(5):R181

[26] Purkayastha S, Sorond F. Transcranial doppler ultrasound: Technique and application. Seminars in Neurology. 2012;**32**(4):411-420

[27] Algebaly H, ElSherbini S, Galal A, Hamdi R, Baz A, Elbeleidy A. Transcranial doppler can predict development and outcome of Sepsis-associated encephalopathy in Pediatrics with severe Sepsis or septic shock. Frontiers in Pediatric. 2020;**2020**:8

[28] Pierrakos C, Attou R, Decorte L, Kolyviras A, Malinverni S, Gottignies P, et al. Transcranial doppler to assess sepsis-associated encephalopathy in critically ill patients. BMC Anesthesiology. 2014;**14**:45

[29] Crippa IA, Subirà C, Vincent JL, Fernandez RF, Hernandez SC, Cavicchi FZ, et al. Impaired cerebral autoregulation is associated with brain dysfunction in patients with

sepsis. Critical Care London English. 2018;**22**(1):327

[30] Sanz D, D'Arco F, Robles CA, Brierley J. Incidence and pattern of brain lesions in paediatric septic shock patients. The British Journal of Radiology. 2018;**91**(1084):20170861

[31] Kim MB, Ward DS, Cartwright CR, Kolano J, Chlebowski S, Henson LC. Estimation of jugular venous O2 saturation from cerebral oximetry or arterial O2 saturation during isocapnic hypoxia. Journal of Clinical Monitoring and Computing. 2000;**16**(3):191-199

[32] McLeod AD, Igielman F, Elwell C, Cope M, Smith M. Measuring cerebral oxygenation during normobaric hyperoxia: A comparison of tissue microprobes, near-infrared spectroscopy, and jugular venous oximetry in head injury. Anesthesia and Analgesia. 2003 Sep;**97**(3):851-856

[33] Taussky P, O'Neal B, Daugherty WP, Luke S, Thorpe D, Pooley RA, et al. Validation of frontal near-infrared spectroscopy as noninvasive bedside monitoring for regional cerebral blood flow in brain-injured patients. Neurosurgical Focus. 2012;**32**(2):E2

[34] Wood M, Song A, Maslove D, Ferri C, Howes D, Muscedere J, et al. Brain tissue oxygenation in patients with septic shock: A feasibility study. The Canadian Journal of Neurological Sciences. 2016;**43**(1):65-73

[35] Scott JP, Hoffman GM. Near-infrared spectroscopy: Exposing the dark (venous) side of the circulation. Paediatric Anaesthesia. 2014;**24**(1):74-88

[36] Marin T, Moore J. Understanding near-infrared spectroscopy. Advanced Neonatal Care Official Journal of National Association Neonatal Nurses. 2011;**11**(6):382-388

[37] Shapiro NI, Arnold R, Sherwin R, O'Connor J, Najarro G, Singh S, et al. The association of near-infrared spectroscopy-derived tissue oxygenation measurements with sepsis syndromes, organ dysfunction and mortality in emergency department patients with sepsis. Critical Care. 2011;**15**(5):R223

[38] Sutter R, Kaplan PW. Clinical and electroencephalographic correlates of acute encephalopathy. Journal of Clinical Neurophysiological. 2013;**30**:443-453. DOI: 10.1097/WNP.0b013e3182a73bc2

[39] Chong DJ, Hirsch LJ. Which EEG patterns warrant treatment in the critically ill? Reviewing the evidence for treatment of periodic epileptiform discharges and related patterns. Journal of Clinical Neurophysiology. 2005;**22**:79-91. DOI: 10.1097/01.wnp.0000158699.78529.af

[40] Kurtz P, Gaspard N, Wahl AS, et al. Continuous electroencephalography in a surgical intensive care unit. Intensive Care Medicine. 2014;**40**:228-234. DOI: 10.1007/s00134-013-3149-8

[41] Hosokawa K, Gaspard N, Su F, Oddo M, Vincent J-L, Taccone FS. Clinical neurophysiological assessment of sepsis-associated brain dysfunction: A systematic review. Critical Care. 2014;**18**:674

[42] Mazeraud A, Righy C, Bouchereau E, Benghanem S, Bozza FA, Sharshar T. Septic-associated encephalopathy: A comprehensive review. Neurotherapeutics. 2020;**17**:392-403

[43] Foreman B, Claassen J, Abou Khaled K, Jirsch J, Alschuler DM, Wittman J, et al. Generalized periodic discharges in the critically ill: A case-control study of 200 patients. Neurology. 2012;**79**:1951-1960

[44] Moruzzi G, Magoun HW. Brain stem reticular formation and activation of the EEG. Electroencephalography and Clinical Neurophysiology. 1949;**1**:455-473

[45] Shehabi Y, Riker RR, Bokesch PM, et al. Delirium duration and mortality in lightly sedated, mechanically ventilated intensive care patients. Critical Care Medicine. 2010;**38**:2311-2318. DOI: 10.1097/CCM.0b013e3181f85759

[46] Oddo M, Carrera E, Claassen J, et al. Continuous electroencephalography in the medical intensive care unit. Critical Care Medicine. 2009;**37**:2051-2056. DOI: 10.1097/CCM.0b013e3181a00604

[47] Duncan CC, Barry RJ, Connolly JF, Fischer C, Michie PT, Näätänen R, et al. Event-related potentials in clinical research: Guidelines for eliciting, recording, and quantifying mismatch negativity, P300, and N400. Clinical Neurophysiological Official Journal. 2009;**120**:1883-1908

[48] Guérit JM. Neurophysiological testing in neurocritical care. Current Opinion in Critical Care. 2010;**16**(2):98-104

[49] Rinaldi S, Consales G, De Gaudio AR. Changes in auditory evoked potentials induced by postsurgical sepsis. Minerva Anestesiologica. 2008;**74**(6):245-250

[50] Sweis R, Ortiz J, Biller J. Neurology of Sepsis. Current Neurology and Neuroscience Reports. 2016;**16**:21

[51] Zauner C, Gendo A, Kramer L, Funk GC, Bauer E, Schenk P, et al. Impaired subcortical and cortical sensory evoked potential pathways in septic patients. Critical Care Medicine. 2002;**30**(5):1136-1139

[52] Savvina IA, Zabrodskaya YuM, Petrova AO. General anesthesia and autonomic nervous system: Control and management in neurosurgery. In: Aslanidis T, Nouris C, editors. Autonomic Nervous System – Special Interest Topics. Vol. 14. IntechOpen Series. London: IntechOpen; 2022. pp. 53-76

[53] Nolan JP, Sandroni C, Böttiger BW, Cariou A, Cronberg T, Friberg H, et al. European resuscitation council and European Society of Intensive Care Medicine guidelines 2021: Post-resuscitation care. Intensive Care Medicine. 2021;**47**(4):369-421

[54] Sandroni C, Cariou A, Cavallaro F, Cronberg T, Friberg H, Hoedemaekers C, et al. Prognostication in comatose survivors of cardiac arrest: An advisory statement from the European resuscitation council and the European Society of Intensive Care Medicine. Intensive Care Medicine. 2014;**40**(12):1816-1831

[55] Joshi S, Li Y, Kalwani RM, Gold JI. Relationships between pupil diameter and neuronal activity in the locus coeruleus, colliculi, and cingulate cortex. Neuron. 2016;**89**(1):221-234

[56] Couret D, Boumaza D, Grisotto C, Triglia T, Pellegrini L, Ocquidant P, et al. Reliability of standard pupillometry practice in neurocritical care: An observational, double-blinded study. Critical Care London English. 2016;**20**:99

[57] Larson MD, Behrends M. Portable infraredpupillometry:Areview.Anesthesia and Analgesic. 2015;**120**(6):1242-1253

[58] Solari D, Rossetti AO, Carteron L, Miroz JP, Novy J, Eckert P, et al. Early prediction of coma recovery after cardiac arrest with blinded pupillometry. Annals of Neurology. 2017;**81**(6):804-810

[59] Tamura T, Namiki J, Sugawara Y, Sekine K, Yo K, Kanaya T, et al.

Quantitative assessment of pupillary light reflex for early prediction of outcomes after out-of-hospital cardiac arrest: A multicentre prospective observational study. Resuscitation. 2018;**131**:108-113

[60] Oddo M, Sandroni C, Citerio G, Miroz JP, Horn J, Rundgren M, et al. Quantitative versus standard pupillary light reflex for early prognostication in comatose cardiac arrest patients: An international prospective multicenter double-blinded study. Intensive Care Medicine. 2018;**44**:2102-2111

[61] Quispe Cornejo A, Fernandes Vilarinho CS, Crippa IA, Peluso L, Calabrò L, Vincent JL, et al. The use of automated pupillometry to assess cerebral autoregulation: A retrospective study. Journal of Intensive Care. 2020;**8**(1):57

[62] Stålberg E, van Dijk H, Falck B, et al. Standards for quantification of EMG and neurography. Clinical Neurophysiology. 2019;**130**(9):1688-1729

[63] Tennilä A, Salmi T, Pettilä V, Roine RO, Varpula T, Takkunen O. Early signs of critical illness polyneuropathy in ICU patients with systemic inflammatory response syndrome or sepsis. Intensive Care Medicine. 2000;**26**(9):1360-1363

[64] Hermans G, Van den Berghe G. Clinical review: Intensive care unit acquired weakness. Critical Care. 2015;**19**(1):274

[65] Latronico N, Bolton CF. Critical illness polyneuropathy and myopathy: A major cause of muscle weakness and paralysis. Lancet Neurology. 2011;**10**:931-941

[66] Stevens RD, Marshall SA, Cornblath DR, et al. A framework for diagnosing and classifying intensive care unit-acquired weakness. Critical Care Medicine. 2009;**37**:S299-S308

[67] Satyapriya SV, Lyaker ML, Rozycki AJ, Papadimos T. Sedation, Analgesia Delirium in the ECMO Patient. Extracorporeal Membrane Oxygenation: Advances in Therapy. Chapter 14. IntechOpen; 2016. pp. 287-304. DOI: 10.5772/64249

Chapter 5

Research Progress on Virulence Factors of *Vibrio alginolyticus*: A Key Pathogenic Bacteria of Sepsis

Hongyan Cai, Jiaying Yu, Qiu Li, Youyu Zhang and Lixing Huang

Abstract

As an opportunistic pathogen, *V. alginolyticus* is commonly found in people with weak immune systems or open wounds. The history of seafood exposure is a major feature of *V. alginolyticus* infection. *V. alginolyticus* can infect marine economic animals such as fish, shrimp, and shellfish, and is also one of the key pathogens that cause sepsis in human. Because of its rapid progress and extremely high mortality after the infection, it has received more and more attention in clinical practice. At present, there is no effective method to completely control the incidence of *V. alginolyticus*. Therefore, it is particularly important to study the virulence factors and pathogenic mechanisms of *V. alginolyticus*. This article reviews recent studies on virulence factors of *V. alginolyticus*, such as quorum sensing, virulence proteins, ferroportin hemolysin, flagella, lipopolysaccharide system and biofilm formation, with the hope of providing further insights into aquaculture and public health.

Keywords: *V. alginolyticus*, sepsis, virulence, molecular mechanism, virulence proteins, flagellar system, hemolysin

1. Introduction

Sepsis is a syndrome in which the host's response to infection is unbalanced. It refers to an acute systemic infection caused by pathogens or opportunistic pathogens that invade the blood circulation, grow and multiply in the blood, and produce toxins, which can lead to life-threatening organ dysfunction [1]. Sepsis, an epidemic disease with acute morbidity and high mortality, accounts for a large portion of global healthcare expenditures each year [2]. If sepsis is not quickly controlled, it will develop from the primary infection site to other parts of the body, causing metastatic abscesses [3], and then causing meningitis, osteomyelitis, arthritis, etc., and finally due to the accumulation of pus anywhere in the body can form an abscess, severe septic shock, and migratory lesions. Sepsis is extremely harmful to humans, and so far, no rapid and effective diagnostic biomarkers or sepsis-targeted therapeutics have been developed [4]. This may be due to the substantial heterogeneity of disease resulting from multiple underlying pathogens, sites of infection, individualized host immune responses, and manifestations of organ dysfunction [5]. Current research shows that the pathogenic *Vibrio* that cause sepsis mainly include *Vibrio vulnificus* [6], *Vibrio cholerae* [7], and *V. alginolyticus* [8]. Among them, *V. alginolyticus*, as an emerging pathogenic bacterium, can infect aquatic animals and humans, which not only seriously affects the quality and safety of aquatic food, but also causes human disease and threatens public health.

V. alginolyticus is a globally distributed opportunistic pathogen and one of the most harmful pathogenic bacteria in marine vibriosis caused by *V. alginolyticus* has also increased, resulting in huge economic loss [9]. In recent years, with the rapid development of aquaculture, the water quality and environment of aquaculture have frequently been polluted and eutrophicated, and the number of vibriosis cases caused by *V. alginolyticus* has also increased, resulting in huge economic losses and impact on the healthy development of the aquaculture industry. *V. alginolyticus*, as one of the most abundant *Vibrio* species in marine *Vibrio*, causes *Vibrio* disease with high morbidity, high mortality and wide prevalence. Infected and then caused host disease [10]. The infection of fish by *V. alginolyticus* will cause septicemia, mainly with symptoms of bleeding, dark skin and ulcers on the skin surface [11]. Aquatic products and drinking water contaminated with *V. alginolyticus* can lead to human infection and disease outbreaks [12]. *V. alginolyticus* can not only contaminate food alone or in combination with other pathogenic bacteria to cause food poisoning, but also cause otitis media, external ear infections Inflammation, gastrointestinal diseases [13–15], etc., especially those with weak immune systems or open wounds are more susceptible to disease. According to research reports, Chien et al. believe that *V. alginolyticus* as the cause of pleural empyema and bacteremia in an immunocompromised patient [8]. Gaüzère et al. believe that *V. alginolyticus* is the pathogen of sepsis in the Indian Ocean, especially those who are engaged in marine activities are most likely to be infected by it and cause sepsis [16]. Li et al. reported the eventual death of a patient with septic shock caused by *V. alginolyticus* infection [17]. It can be seen that *V. alginolyticus* is one of the key pathogenic bacteria of sepsis.

In order to meet the diverse needs of human food, the mariculture industry is booming around the world, but the economic losses caused by vibriosis make the mariculture industry face huge challenges. *V. alginolyticus* can infect human body and fish and induce disease, causing great harm to human health and mariculture. Disease mechanism. Although *V. alginolyticus* is sensitive to most antibiotics, it is highly resistant to antibiotics such as penicillin, erythromycin, vancomycin, ampicillin, sulfisoxazole, and sulfonamides [15, 18, 19]. Shahimi [20] et al. identified the presence of four antibiotic resistance genes for penicillin (*pbp2a*), ampicillin (*blaOXA*), erythromycin (*ermB*) and vancomycin (*vanB*) by polymerase chain reaction. This is also one of the reasons for the repeated infection of *V. alginolyticus* in mariculture, which is difficult to treat, with wide damage area, long disease course and high mortality. With the increasingly strict restrictions on the use of antibiotics in modern aquaculture, there is no effective method to completely control the incidence of *V. alginolyticus*, so it is particularly important to study the virulence factors and pathogenic mechanism of the bacteria.

The pathogenic process of *V. alginolyticus* on the host body is complex and diverse. First, it adheres to the surface of host cells through adhesion. Adhesion plays a decisive role in invading host cells and causing disease. In the end, the products of its growth and metabolism contain toxins, which will directly interfere and destroy the metabolism and function of the host body [21]. This series of pathogenic processes of *V. alginolyticus* occurs under the combined action of its own environment, virulence determinants and the living conditions of the host [22, 23], in which the virulence factor is the main manifestation of the pathogenicity of *V. alginolyticus*, and its intensity is jointly determined by the invasiveness, infectivity and pathogenicity. At present, efforts have been done to understand the pathogenic mechanism and regulatory system of *V. alginolyticus*. The main researches are about the quorum sensing system (QS) [24], virulence protein [25, 26], siderophore [27], adhesion [28], flagellar system, hemolysin and biofilm formation [29], etc. However, the specific molecular mechanism of the pathogenicity of *V. alginolyticus* virulence regulation has not been fully illustrated.

Multi-omics is the combined application of a variety of high-throughput omics technologies, mainly including gene/transcriptomics [30], proteomics [31], metabolomics [32], as well as epigenetics [33]. It is a technology that comprehensively analyzes information to clarify a certain biological mechanism. In recent years, multiomics technologies have developed rapidly in fields such as life sciences and medicine, but each individual technology cannot capture the overall view of a biological mechanism, and comprehensive multiomics analysis may be able to reveal new insights. With the rapid application of multiomics in the detection and analysis of biological samples, the reduction of time and cost required to generate these datasets, omics datasets bring both opportunities and challenges for scientists. The present review will focus on comparative analysis of advances in genomics, transcriptomics, proteomics and metabolomics in the study of the molecular mechanism of pathogenicity of *V. alginolyticus* virulence regulation, providing new opportunities to identify new targets to help us understanding the pathogenic mechanism of *V. alginolyticus*. Here, we review recent findings based on multi-omics studies of virulence factor-related genes/proteins in *V. alginolyticus*, and provide an in-depth summary of our current understanding of the pathogenic mechanisms of *V. alginolyticus*. This review also provides guidance and suggestions for basic research and innovative perspectives on pathogenic mechanisms of *V. alginolyticus* virulence factors.

1.1 Quorum sensing system

Quorum sensing is a communication process between bacterial cells. Bacteria sense changes in population cell density by measuring the concentration of extracellular autoinducers [34]. In 1979, Nealson et al. first discovered quorum sensing in the bioluminescent marine bacterium *Vibrio fischeri* and found that quorum sensing has the function of regulating bacterial bioluminescence [35]. The bacterial population produces a certain amount of signal molecules through background expression and transports them out of the cell. With the increase of bacterial cell density, the concentration of signal molecules will also increase. When the concentration of signal molecules in the surrounding environment reaches a threshold, the QS will be triggered. The QS is an important regulatory system for the expression of *Vibrio* virulence. In the QS system of *V. alginolyticus*, LuxR and AphA homologous proteins are the two main central regulatory elements (MQSRs) that control gene expression [36]. This system mainly transmits the cell density signal in the form of phosphate groups through the AIs histidine kinase receptor into the cell, and then transmits it to the regulatory protein LuxO step by step. The phosphorylation state of LuxO determines whether Qrrs is expressed. Under the action of Hfq, Qrrs mainly regulates the expression of MQSR proteins (AphA and LuxR homologous proteins) and regulates the expression of QS pathway and QS-related biological pathway genes. AphA and LuxR homologous proteins jointly regulate 99% of the genes in the QS regulatory element [34, 37], while the rest of the genes are post-transcriptionally regulated by Qrrs

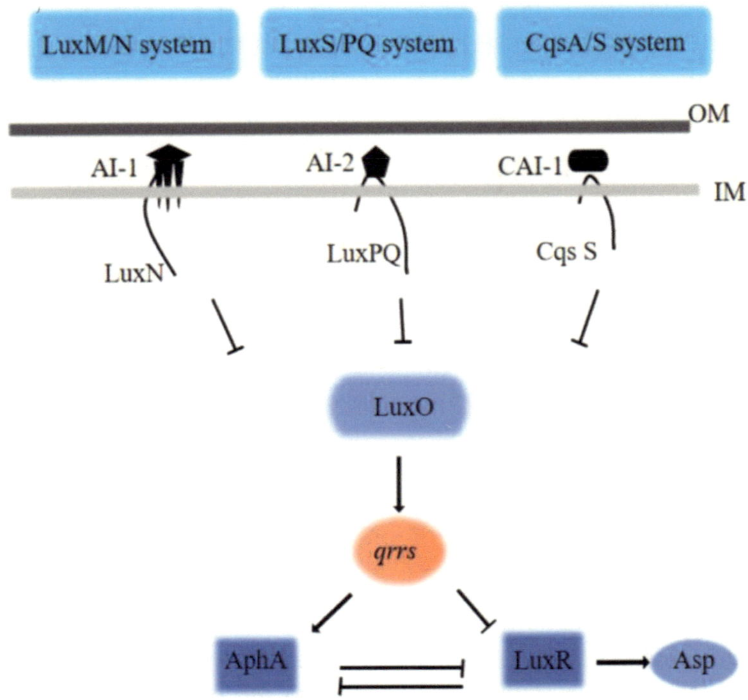

Figure 1.
Quorum sensing system of Vibrio alginolyticus.

(**Figure 1**) [38]. Therefore, in this QS system, AphA and LuxR homologous proteins are considered as central regulatory elements of quorum sensing, and their regulatory functions are conserved in *V. alginolyticus*.

In the quorum sensing system of *V. alginolyticus*, LuxR is involved in the regulation of high cell density (HCD) stage, while AphA is involved in the regulation of gene expression in low cell density (LCD) stage. AphA regulates the expression of multiple genes, especially those encoding virulence factors, flagella, motility, and biofilm formation [39, 40]. AphA negatively regulates the expression of the major virulence factor alkaline serine protease (Asp) through LuxR. Gu et al. [40] detected 49 sites rich in AphA binding peaks in the genome of *V. alginolyticus* by chromatin immuno-precipitation (ChIP) and high-throughput DNA sequencing (ChIP-seq) technology. It was demonstrated that AphA can directly regulate genes encoding adenylate cyclase (anti-σD, FabR and small RNA CsrB). At the same time, it was also revealed that AphA regulates motility through the coordinated function of LuxR and CsrB. Liu et al. [41] verified the existence of cell density-dependent sRNA Qrr in *V. alginolyticus* by transcriptomics and was homologous to QS-regulated sRNA Qrr1-5. Qrr is mainly produced under LCD and regulates the master regulators LuxR and AphA in the quorum sensing (QS) pathway at the post-transcriptional level. And both LuxR and AphA can directly bind to the promoter of qrr to activate or repress its transcription, respectively. Zhen et al. [42] found through phosphorylation proteomic studies that VstR phosphorylated by *V. alginolyticus* can enhance the expression of LuxR, thereby inhibiting T6SS1 or promoting the activity of T6SS2. In addition, the phosphatase PppA can affect the activity of QS by regulating the transcription level of LuxR, thereby regulating the expression of hcp and vgrG3 operons in T6SS.

In addition to LuxR and AphA, a third MQSR, VqsA, was found in *V. alginolyticus* through transcriptomic studies. This protein is a new LysR family transcription factor, which can regulate the biofilm formation of *V. alginolyticus*, the production of exotoxin Asp, the bactericidal ability mediated by T6SS2, and the pathogenicity to fish by directly activating LuxR and inhibiting the expression of AphA [43]. The VqsA protein shares a similar C-terminal ligand-binding domain with another LysR family protein, AphB, which is considered to be a key virulence regulator in *V. alginolyticus*. Through structural analysis, it was found that Cys189 and Cys166 may have a similar function to the thiol switch Cys235 of AphB protein, which can respond to acid stress and oxidative stress [44]. The three MQSR proteins, LuxR, AphA and VqsA, all inhibit their own expression while regulating each other, which further shows the complex regulatory network and function mediated by these factors in V. alginolyticus [43–45].

In the QS system of *V. alginolyticus*, LuxO-LuxR regulation is closely related to its virulence, by cloning another novel regulator luxT [46]. Transcription of the luxT gene is cell density-dependent, and is positively regulated by LuxU and characterized in the QS cascade to play multiple roles in regulating ECP production and motility in *V. alginolyticus*. At the same time, a new pathway, luxT, which is completely different from *Vibrio harveyi* and *Vibrio vulnificus*, was also discovered in *V. alginolyticus*. luxT can activate luxO expression at the transcriptional level as well as luxR expression at the post-transcriptional level [47]. The AhpA and LuxR proteins of *V. alginolyticus* are extremely important central regulatory elements in the quorum sensing system, and have a close regulatory relationship with virulence factors and metabolic pathways. Therefore, it is of great significance to search for regulated transcriptional regulators.

1.2 Biofilm mechanism

Most pathogenic bacteria do not exist in a single cell and planktonic state in the host's internal environment, but in the form of a group biofilm. The discovery of

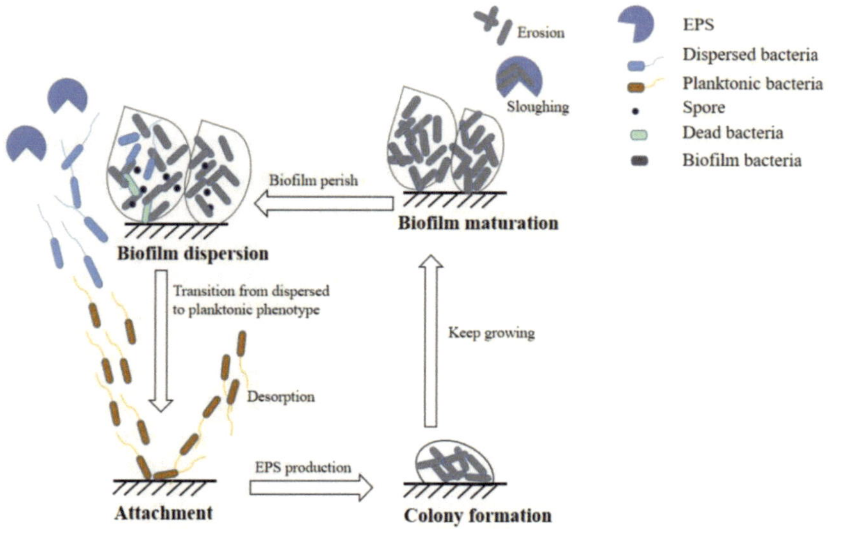

Figure 2.
Biofilm development process.

bacterial biofilms can be traced back to 1676 when Leeuwenhoek observed biofilms from his own dental plaque, but it was not a cause for concern at the time. It was not until 1978 that Costerton and others proposed the related concept of biofilm and reported the pathogenicity and drug resistance of bacterial biofilm, and the cell membrane attracted the attention of scholars [48, 49]. BF is a bacteria adhesion to the surface of inert or active objects, and surrounded by polysaccharide matrix, protein, lipids and other extracellular matrices (EPS), forming a highly organized, systematic membrane-like polymer with a special complex structure [50]. BF formation is a dynamic process closely related to exopolysaccharide production, cell migration, subpopulation differentiation and interactions (**Figure 2**). Studies show that the formation process of BF of *V. alginolyticus* mainly includes four processes: (i) Bacteria attach to biotic or abiotic surfaces; (ii) Bacteria lose their ability to move and begin to produce biofilm substrates, forming biofilms; (iii) Biofilm maturation and thickening; (iv) Biofilm diffusion (with the aging of the biofilm, bacteria disperse from the biofilm and revert to a planktonic state, and the life cycle begins again) [51, 52].

Bacterial biofilms are an important mechanism leading to bacterial resistance and are associated with most bacterial infections. According to CDC statistics, 65% of human bacterial infections are related to the formation of biofilms [53]. Biofilms make bacteria in biofilms significantly more resistant to antibiotics and disinfectants than planktonic bacteria through a series of different mechanisms. For example, the impermeability of the biofilm matrix to antibiotics, the reduced growth rate of bacteria at the core of the biofilm, the presence of antibiotic-resistant persister bacteria, and the overexpression of bacterial efflux pumps in the biofilm, causing persistent infection, are the main reasons for treatment failure [54]. RpoN has been reported to be involved in *Vibrio* biofilm formation, and RpoN (σ54) acts as a global regulator to control key virus-associated phenotypes, which can regulate flagella and extracellular polysaccharides (EPS) during pathogenic biofilm formation. Zhang et al. showed that when the *rpoN* gene in *Vibrio alginolyticus* is deleted, it will lead to the failure of biofilm detachment, the loss of flagella and the reduction of motility, which proves that *rpoN* is crucial for the separation of *V. alginolyticus* biofilms [55]. Gu et al. concluded through RNA-seq and ChIP-seq that RpoE and RpoX have different regulators, regulating a total of 105 genes under high temperature conditions, including those related to biofilm formation, motility, virulence and other related genes, meanwhile, it was proved that RpoX can up-regulate genes related to flagella, biofilm formation and hemolytic activity at higher temperature [56].

Some studies have found [57, 58] that bacterial biofilm formation is closely related to its swarm effect, and swarm effect mutants cannot form normal mature biofilm structures, and their resistance to drugs and host immune systems is significantly reduced. Stringent responses mediated by the bacterial alarmins pppGpp and ppGpp [collectively (p)ppGpp] are considered important adaptive responses to stressful conditions. Yin Wenliang et al. showed that in *V. alginolyticus*, the (p)ppGpp synthase genes *relA* and *spoT* can contribute to biofilm formation at low cell density and biofilm formation at high cell density, respectively. It was also shown that (p)ppGpp could serve as a key regulator of *V. alginolyticus* biofilm formation [59]. As a three-phase ATP-independent periplasmic transporter solute-binding subunit, DctP. Zhang et al. constructed a *dctp* mutant strain, compared with the wild strain of *V. alginolyticus*, its biofilm formation ability was significantly reduced. Further transcriptomic analysis showed that the deletion mutation of *dctp* could regulate the expression levels of 22 related genes in the colonization, adhesion and pathogenicity of *V. alginolyticus* [60]. Oligopeptide permease (Opp) has now been shown to play an important role in the virulence of *V. alginolyticus*. Liu et al. identified the *opp* gene cluster in the transcriptome sequence of *V. alginolyticus*, and proved that *oppABCDF* has an important contribution to the biofilm formation of *V. alginolyticus*, among which *oppA* and *oppB* have the greatest influence, and *oppF* has the minimal impact [29]. The *toxR* is a conserved virulence-related gene in *Vibrio*. Chen et al. found that the deletion of *toxR* can significantly reduce the biofilm formation ability of *V. alginolyticus*. The analysis of outer membrane protein (OMP) showed that ToxR may enhance the formation of biofilm by regulating the production of OMP [61]. In addition, EPS can immobilize microbial communities in biofilms and maintain a series of highly complex dynamic changes that play important roles in both biofilm structure and function, including surface adhesion, spatial and chemical heterogeneity, biofilm virulence composition, attenuates the effects of antimicrobial agents, and promotes cell-to-cell interactions, thereby enhancing the metabolic capacity and drug resistance of cells in biofilms [62].

Due to different microbial species, local shear stress, nutrient and substrate utilization, and host environment, biofilm EPS matrix composition and structure are quite different [50]; moreover, the secretion and spatial organization of EPS also differ between single and multiple bacterial communities [62]. Microbial species and metabolic activity, nutrient availability, host environment, and growth stage all affect the variability of EPS composition and structure, making it difficult to develop EPS-targeting drugs and technologies. Various EPS substrates secreted by *V. alginolyticus* play important roles in maintaining the stability and scaffolding of biofilm structures, and are also involved in biofilm assembly, population behavior, and functional properties of toxicity, such as signaling, genetic exchange, microenvironment formation, mechanical stability, antibiotic resistance, etc. Although some studies have revealed the composition and function of EPS matrix in the biofilm system of some model microorganisms, the underlying mechanisms of complex signaling molecules and biofilm formation and virulence factor expression still need to be elucidated.

1.3 Siderophore system

Iron is an essential element for the pathogenic process of *V. alginolyticus* and plays an important role in the life activity of *V. alginolyticus*. Although iron is abundant in nature, in the host body it is usually bound to proteins to form complexes, and the level of iron ions free outside the cells is very low [63, 64]. In order to obtain iron in the host, pathogenic pathogens such as *V. alginolyticus* have developed two iron uptake systems, one that destroys erythrocytes in host tissues through exotoxins and then obtains iron ions from heme released from erythrocytes, and the other that produces high-affinity iron carriers (siderophores) that can transport iron taken up from transferrin and lactoferrin to bacteriophage cells for their own use through transport [63].

The ability to take up available dissolved iron ions from the environment is essential for the growth of most bacteria in an iron-limited environment. In bacteria, iron uptake mechanisms undertaken by iron carriers have evolved for this purpose. Genes for the synthesis and transport of iron carriers are usually present in chromosomes or plasmids. Two groups of enzymes, non-ribosomal peptide synthase (NRPS) and NRPS-independent synthase (NIS) [65], are responsible for iron carrier biosynthesis [66]. In Gram-negative bacteria, the iron-iron carrier complex is recognized by speciWc tonb-activated outer membrane receptors and then transferred to successive components, such as periplasmic binding proteins and permease proteins [67]. In most cases, the expression of genes required for the synthesis and transport of iron carriers is readily regulated by a combination of biologically effective iron concentrations and iron uptake regulatory proteins (Fur) to maintain optimal intracellular iron growth at a relatively stable concentration [68]. Among other pathogenic *Vibrio* species, the strong iron carrier-mediated iron acquisition system is considered to be one of the important virulence advantages [69].

Wang et al. [27] isolated from the pathogenic bacterium Vibrio MVP01, a cluster of 11 genes consisting of two differentially transcribed manipulators pvsABCDE and psuA-pvuABCDE, regulated by Fe^{3+} and iron uptake regulators (Fur), with high similarity to loci associated with iron carrier biosynthesis and transport in *Vibrio parahaemolyticus*. When single in-frame mutations occur in *pvsA* and *pvsD* of the *pvsABCDE* manipulator or *pvuA, pvuB* and *pvuE* of the *psuA-pvuABCDE* manipulator, they prevent the biosynthesis or utilization of algal iron carriers, indicating that they play an important role in the biosynthesis or utilization of iron carriers in *V. alginolyticus* MVP01. Addition of purified iron carriers restored cell growth of iron carrier biosynthesis mutants, but not iron carrier uptake mutants [27]. Wang et al. [24] cloned the *luxO* gene from *V. alginolyticus* MVP01 through genomic studies, and gene analysis showed that it encodes a protein highly similar to other LuxO homologs. *luxO* in-frame deletion mutants and *rpoN* null mutants were constructed with suicide plasmids, demonstrating that deletion of LuxO alone increased extracellular protease and hemolysis product secretion, but reduced *V. alginolyticus* MVP01 production of iron carriers. The *rpoN* deletion mutants showed significantly higher protease levels and iron carrier production, and significantly lower hemolytic activity of ECP. *V. alginolyticus* has a functional *luxO* gene that regulates the secretion of extracellular proteases and hemolytic substances and the production of iron carriers in an r54-dependent or independent manner. *V. alginolyticus* MVP01 produces extracellular proteases and hemolytic active substances as well as iron carriers, which may characterize the virulence of this strain. Uncovering the regulation of the secretion of these products by LuxO and r54 and the potential population sensing system of *V. alginolyticus* MVP01 will contribute to the understanding of the pathogenesis of *Vibrio* [24].

1.4 Flagellar system

Bacterial motility is a mechanism shared by many microorganisms and is necessary for pathogenic bacteria to invade their hosts and achieve their life activities; therefore, it is treated as an important virulence factor for many pathogens [70], and the flagellum is one of the main motility organs of bacteria, while the number and location of flagella vary depending on the bacterial species [71]. *V. alginolyticus* contains two unique flagellar systems, (i) a polar flagellum with a membrane sheath suitable for swimming in a liquid environment and (ii) a large number of lateral flagella suitable for aggregation on the surface of living and nonliving objects and produced only when the polar flagellum is not functional [72, 73].

The LuxS population sensing system has been reported to regulate the expression of several virulence factors of pathogenic bacteria. Inactive *luxS* results in reduced virulence of *V. alginolyticus*. A *luxS*-deficient mutant presents a defect in motility and flagellogenesis, which is compensated by intact *luxS*. Since motility depends on flagella, genes related to *V. alginolyticus* flagellogenesis, including flagellar regulatory genes *flaK* and *lafK* and secondary flagellar genes *fliS* and *lafA*, were cloned and characterized by real-time fluorescence quantitative reverse transcription polymerase. The differential expression of these genes in wild-type and *luxS* mutants was confirmed by real-time fluorescence quantitative reverse transcription polymerase chain reaction. The results indicate that LuxS plays an important regulatory role in motility and flagellar biogenesis in *V. alginolyticus* [74], and the study of the role of *luxS* in kinetic regulation is important for understanding the virulence mechanism of *V. alginolyticus*.

V. alginolyticus usually has unipolar flagella whose number and position are positively regulated by FlhF. Shota Kondo et al. [75] introduced random mutations into FlhF through genomics in mutants that fail to produce flagella at the cell pole, and these new mutations were localized only to the GTPase motif of FlhF. Compared to wild type, mutant FlhF proteins have reduced polar localization and can still bind to membranes. The results suggest that the GTPase motif of FlhF plays a key role in the polar localization of the protein during flagellar formation.

FlhF is a GTPase that is a homolog of the signal recognition particle (SRP) protein Ffh and the SRP receptor FtsY. FlhF is located at the cell poles and directs flagellum formation. FlhF and FlhG are proteins that control flagellum formation in bacteria with flagella at both cell poles [76–78]. *flhF* is involved in determining the location of flagellum formation [79, 80]. *V. alginolyticus* has only one flagellum at the cell pole, and FlhF overexpression or FlhG deficiency leads to the formation of multiple flagella at the cell pole. When FlhF is deficient or FlhG is overexpressed in the cell, the cell has no flagellum. Thus, FlhF and FlhG negatively and positively control the number of flagella, respectively. Furthermore, co-expression of FlhF and FlhG reduces the number of polar flagella more than FlhG alone, suggesting that FlhG co-regulates the number of polar flagella with FlhF. To investigate the interaction between FlhF and FlhG, Akiko Kusumoto et al. [80], using anti-FlhF antibodies for immunoprecipitation, proposed a model in which the localization of FlhF at the pole determines the polar position and flagellar production, and FlhG interacts with FlhF to prevent FlhF from polar positioning, and thus FlhG negatively regulates the number of flagella in *V. alginolyticus* cells.

Zhu [81] et al. studied the sheath flagellum of *V. alginolyticus* by a combination of cryoelectron tomography (cryo ET) and subspectral analysis as well as genetic methods, revealing significant differences between *V. alginolyticus* cells with and without sheath flagella, which have a ring-like structure at the base of the hook that is associated with major remodeling of the outer membrane and sheath formation.

1.5 Hemolysin

Hemolysin, an exotoxin that lyses the erythrocyte membrane by releasing hemoglobin, is the most widely distributed toxin in pathogenic *Vibrio* [82]. Hemolysin acts on the erythrocyte membrane, leading to cell lysis, which in turn releases iron-binding proteins, such as hemoglobin, transferrin and lactoferrin. Iron can then be obtained through a high-affinity iron acquisition system capable of competing with host iron-binding proteins. The main system centers on iron carriers, which are low molecular weight chelators that specifically bind extracellular Fe^{3+} and are subsequently taken up through receptors on the cell membrane [83–85]. Hemolysin expression in Vibrio maritimus is regulated under iron-limited conditions and occurs in the host during infection [84]. In many cases, the hemolysin pore-forming activity is not limited to erythrocytes, but extends to a wide range of other cell types, including mast cells, neutrophils and polymorphonuclear cells, and enhances toxicity by causing tissue damage [86]. There are five representative families of hemolysins in Vibrio, including the heat-resistant direct hemolysin (TDH) family, the HlyA (or E1 Tor hemolysin) family, the heat-resistant hemolysin (TLH) family, the heat-resistant hemolysin (δ-VPH) family, and the novel hemolysin gene (HLX) family [87].

TDH and HlyA have been extensively studied and are closely associated with virulence [87, 88]. However, the role of some other hemolysins, such as TLH, δ-VPH and HLX, is unknown and needs to be determined by further studies.

1.6 Virulence proteins

V. alginolyticus can resist environmental and host-killing effects in many ways. Biofilm formation is one of the important ways. Biofilm formation can enhance host damage by secreting extracellular virulent proteases and exotoxins [89]. At present, the research on the pathogenic mechanism of *V. alginolyticus* has been widely carried out, which is similar to the pathogenic factors of *V. parahaemolyticus* [90]. Its pathogenicity involves many virulence factors, such as heat-resistant direct hemolysin protein (TDH), heat-resistant related hemolysin protein (TRH), type three secretion system (T3SS) and type three secretion system effectors (T3SES) [91, 92].

Studies have shown that the virulence of *V. alginolyticus* is related to the extracellular protease genes *proA* and *vacB*, hemolysin genes *tlh*, *tdh* and *trh*, iron uptake system-related genes tonB-exbB-exbD and density sensing genes *luxO*, *luxS* and *luxR* [93]. Cheng Haiyan studied the virulence-related genes of *toxR* and *acfA*, but the effects of *toxR* and *acfA* genes on the expression of major virulence proteins were not significant [94]. Quan Taishu reported that the same hemolysin TDH as *V. parahaemolyticus* was detected from *V. alginolyticus*, and 86. 0% of the existing strains were positive in Kanagawa test, which proved that the pathogenicity of *V. alginolyticus* was similar to that of *V. parahaemolyticus* [95].

Most of these virulence factors exist in the form of protein, which injects toxin proteins into the host body through the transmembrane transport organs of *vibrio*, such as the secretion system and the two-component system, thus leading to the disease of the body [96]. The type III secretion system is a tightly controlled virulence mechanism that is used for colonization by many Gram-negative bacteria. T3SS consists of cytoplasmic bulbs, a matrix spanning the inner and outer membranes of the cell membrane, and extracellular needles. When infecting the host, T3SS can secrete the virulent protein to the outside of the cell or the surface of the host cell, and even directly "inject" into the host cell and finally cause the death of the host cell [97]. Effector proteins or virulence proteins, the embodiment of bacterial virulence, are directly secreted out of cells or transported to host cells. At present, studies on effector proteins of *V. alginolyticus* type III secretion system are rare. Pang et al. constructed Δ*hopPmaJ*. Compared with wild strains, the virulence, adhesion and swimming ability of Δ*hopPmaJ* were significantly decreased [98]. Zhou et al. constructed Δ*typeA*, which exhibited a significantly reduced toxicity to zebrafish compared with wild strains. Analysis showed that Δ*typeA* could enhance the expression of immune genes such as IgM and IL-1β in fish. It could be demonstrated that by regulating the expression of T3SS gene, it affected the secretion and transport of its effector protein, thereby affecting the pathogenicity of vibrio [98, 99].

1.7 LPS system

LPS is the main component of cell wall, which consists of three parts: core polysaccharide, lipid A and O-specific side chain, and mainly exists in gram-negative bacteria [100, 101]. Among them, lipid A is the toxic part of LPS, which can cause non-specific physiological and pathological reactions in the host, such as fever, disseminated intravascular coagulation, hypotension, leukocyte reaction, and shock. At the same time, LPS is also involved in the process of bacterial adhesion, invasion, and host cell diffusion [102].

Jian et al. immunized grouper with *V. alginolyticus* LPS, and found that LPS can stimulate fish to produce good humoral immune response, and can also significantly improve the activity of lysozyme, antibacterial activity and SOD in experimental fish serum [103]. Therefore, *V. alginolyticus* LPS can be used as a good immunogen, and can also be used as an immunopotentiator to improve the anti-infection ability of fish, which can play an important role in preventing and treating fish diseases. Yan et al. used the lipopolysaccharide solution freeze-dried powder separated from *V. alginolyticus* solution to inject the large yellow croaker with the injection concentration of 0.5 mg/ml. The large yellow croaker died within 5 days. When the concentration was increased to 2 mg/ml, the mortality of the large yellow croaker reached 100% within 3 days [104]. Xu et al. injected lipopolysaccharide of *V. alginolyticus* with different concentrations into *Epinephelus coioides*. The experimental results showed that the immunogenicity of LPS of *V. alginolyticus* on *E. coioides* was enhanced with the increase of LPS concentration, and the immunogenicity of *E. coioides* was also enhanced [105, 106].

It has been found that LPS plays a very important role in the pathogenesis of infection [107]. Zhou et al. studied the structure of Lipid A of *V. parahaemolyticus* and related genes. By gene comparison, they found that there were four genes in *V. parahaemolyticus* ATCC33846 that might be related to the secondary acylation during the synthesis of LIPID A: VP_RS01045, VP_RS00880, VP_RS08405 and VP_RS12170, which provides a further research direction for further research on the structure of the lipopolysaccharide Lipid A of *V. alginolyticus* [108].

2. Conclusions

To sum up, the infection of *V. alginolyticus* is the result of the joint action of multiple virulence factors, which is in line with the general mechanism of pathogenic bacteria. *V. alginolyticus* can cause damage to the tissues of the organism during the invasion and proliferation of the host, and the metabolites produced in this process can further damage the organism or disturb the normal metabolism of the host organism, thereby causing serious outbreaks of diseases in aquatic animals and humans. *V. alginolyticus* infection can range from mild gastroenteritis to necrotizing soft tissue infection, followed by sepsis. For a long time, the prevention and treatment of *Vibrio* disease has been a worldwide problem. Although the use of antibiotics to prevent and control *V. alginolyticus* has certain results, the long-term abuse of antibiotics or drugs will pollute the water environment and lead to the emergence of drug-resistant strains, making the disease control more difficult. Therefore, studying the pathogenic mechanism of septicemia caused by *V. alginolyticus* can provide a relatively comprehensive understanding of *V. alginolyticus*.

Although some known virulence factors of *V. alginolyticus* have been identified, the mechanism of sepsis caused by *V. alginolyticus* remains unclear, and individuals infected with *V. alginolyticus* are still at high risk of sepsis. Combined with the current development trend, the use of gene sequencing and quantitative proteomics, high-throughput screening technology and bioinformatics analysis to identify the potential pathogenic genes and virulence factors of *V. alginolyticus* will be the future research direction.

Author details

Hongyan Cai[1], Jiaying Yu[1], Qiu Li[1], Youyu Zhang[2] and Lixing Huang[1*]

1 Fisheries College, Key Laboratory of Healthy Mariculture for the East China Sea, Ministry of Agriculture, Jimei University, Xiamen, Fujian, PR China

2 Institute of Electromagnetics and Acoustics, School of Electronic Science and Engineering, Xiamen University, Xiamen, Fujian, PR China

*Address all correspondence to: lixinghuang@outlook.com

References

[1] Rudd KE, Kissoon N, Limmathurotsakul D, Bory S, Mutahunga B, Seymour CW, et al. The global burden of sepsis: Barriers and potential solutions. Critical Care. 2018;**22**(1):1-11

[2] Reyes M, Filbin MR, Bhattacharyya RP, Billman K, Eisenhaure T, Hung DT, et al. An immune-cell signature of bacterial sepsis. Nature Medicine. 2020;**26**(3):333-340

[3] Reducing the global burden of sepsis: A positive legacy for the COVID-19 pandemic? Intensive Care Medicine. 2021:733-736

[4] Filbin MR, Lynch J, Gillingham TD, Thorsen JE, Pasakarnis CL, Nepal S, et al. Presenting symptoms independently predict mortality in septic shock: Importance of a previously unmeasured confounder. Critical Care Medicine. 2018;**46**(10):1592-1599

[5] Seymour CW, Kennedy JN, Wang S, Chang CCH, Elliott CF, Xu Z, et al. Derivation, validation, and potential treatment implications of novel clinical phenotypes for sepsis. JAMA. 2019;**321**(20):2003-2017

[6] Sheer AJ, Kline KP, Lo MC. From sea to bloodstream: Vibrio vulnificus sepsis. The American Journal of Medicine. 2017;**130**(10):1167-1169

[7] Shashindran N, Narendrakumar L, Udayakumaran S, Vijayakumar DM, Thomas S, Kumar A. First report of Vibrio cholerae O9, novel st520, isolated from a child with bacteraemia-associated sepsis. Indian Journal of Medical Microbiology. 2020;**38**(3-4):489-491

[8] Chien J, Shih J, Hsueh P, Yang P, Luh K. Vibrio alginolyticus as the cause of pleural empyema and bacteremia in an immunocompromised patient. European Journal of Clinical Microbiology and Infectious Diseases. 2002;**21**(5):401

[9] Colwell RR, Grimes DJ. Vibrio diseases of marine fish populations. Helgoländer Meeresuntersuchungen. 1984;**37**(1-4):265-287

[10] Cai SH, Huang YC, Lu YS, Wu ZH, Wang B, Tang JF, et al. Expression and immunogenicity analysis of accessory colonization factor A from Vibrio alginolyticus strain HY9901. Fish & Shellfish Immunology. 2013;**34**(2):454-462

[11] Lee KK. Pathogenesis studies on Vibrio alginolyticus in the grouper, Epinephelus malabaricus, Bloch et Schneider. Microb Pathog. 19 Jul 1995;**19**(1):39-48

[12] Wentworth, Berttina B. "Diagnostic procedures for bacterial infections." Diagnostic procedures for bacterial infections. 1987;868-868

[13] Prieto JR, Palazón JH. Otitis media due to Vibrio alginolyticus: The risks of the Mediterranean Sea. Anales Espanoles de Pediatria. 1993;**39**(4):361-363

[14] Ardiç N, Ozyurt M. Case report: Otitis due to Vibrio alginolyticus. Mikrobiyoloji Bulteni. 2004;**38**(1-2):145-148

[15] Mukherji A, Schroeder S, Deyling C, Procop GW. An unusual source of vibrio alginolyticus–associated otitis: Prolonged colonization or freshwater exposure? Archives of Otolaryngology–Head & Neck Surgery. 2000;**126**(6):790-791

[16] Gaüzère BA, Chanareille P, Vandroux D. Post nearly drowning Vibrio

alginolyticus septicemia acquired in reunion (Indian Ocean). Bulletin de la Societe de Pathologie Exotique (1990). 2016;**109**(3):151-154

[17] Lee DY, Moon SY, Lee SO, Yang HY, Lee HJ, Lee MS. Septic shock due to Vibrio alginolyticus in a cirrhotic patient: the first case in Korea. Yonsei Medical Journal. 2008;**49**(2):329-332

[18] Menezes FGD, Rodriguez MT, Carvalho FCD, Rebouças RH, Costa RA. Pathogenic Vibrio species isolated from estuarine environments (Ceará, Brazil)-antimicrobial resistance and virulence potential profiles. Anais da Academia Brasileira de Ciências. 2017;**89**:1175-1188

[19] Damir K, Irena VS, Damir V, Emin T. Occurrence, characterization and antimicrobial susceptibility of Vibrio alginolyticus in the Eastern Adriatic Sea. Marine Pollution Bulletin. 2013;**75**(1-2):46-52

[20] Shahimi S, Elias A, Salami M, Fauzi F, Ghani A, Azuhairi A. Antibiotic resistance and determination of resistant genes among cockle (Anadara granosa) isolates of Vibrio alginolyticus. Environmental Science and Pollution Research. 2021;**28**(32):44002-44013

[21] Huang L, Hu J, Su Y, et al. Identification and characterization of three V. *alginolyticus* non-coding RNAs involved in adhesion, chemotaxis, and motility processes. Frontiers in Cellular and Infection Microbiology. 2015;**5**:56

[22] Lee KK, Yu SR, Yang TI, et al. Isolation and characterization of V. alginolyticus isolated from diseased kuruma prawn, Penaeus japonicus. Letters in Applied Microbiology. 1996;**22**(2):111-114

[23] Bejarano PA, Langeveld JP, Hudson BG, et al. Degradation of basement membranes by Pseudomonas aeruginosa elastase. Infection and Immunity. 1989;**57**(12):3783-3787

[24] Wang Q, Liu Q, Ma Y, Rui H, Zhang Y. LuxO controls extracellular protease, haemolytic activities and siderophore production in fish pathogen Vibrio alginolyticus. Journal of Applied Microbiology. 2007;**103**(5):1525-1534

[25] Balebona MC, Andreu MJ, Bordas MA, Zorrilla I, Moriñigo MA, Borrego JJ. Pathogenicity of Vibrio alginolyticus for cultured gilt-head sea bream (Sparus aurata L.). Applied and environmental microbiology. 1998;**64**(11):4269-4275

[26] He H, Wang Q, Sheng L, Liu Q, Zhang Y. Functional characterization of Vibrio alginolyticus twin-arginine translocation system: its roles in biofilm formation, extracellular protease activity, and virulence towards fish. Current Microbiology. 2011;**62**(4):1193-1199

[27] Wang Q, Liu Q, Ma Y, Zhou L, Zhang Y. Isolation, sequencing and characterization of cluster genes involved in the biosynthesis and utilization of the siderophore of marine fish pathogen Vibrio alginolyticus. Archives of Microbiology. 2007;**188**(4):433-439

[28] Luo G, Huang L, Su Y, et al. flrA, flrB and flrC regulate adhesion by controlling the expression of critical virulence genes in V. alginolyticus. Emerging Microbes & Infections. 2016;**5**(8)e00511

[29] Liu W, Huang L, Su Y, et al. Contributions of the oligopeptide permeases in multistep of V. alginolyticus pathogenesis. MicrobiologyOpen. 2017;**6**(5):e00511

[30] Beer BK. Bethesda, and biology: How "genomics" came into being. Journal of the National Cancer Institute. 1998;**90**(2):93

[31] Celis JE, Rasmussen HH, Gromov P, et al. The human keratinocyte two-dimensional gel protein database (update 1995): Mapping components of signal transduction pathways. Electrophoresis. 1995;**16**(1):2177-2240

[32] Nicholson JK, Lindon JC. Systems biology: Metabonomics. Nature. 2008;**455**(7216):1054-1056

[33] Hong YU. Epigenetics: Advances of non-coding RNAs regulation in mammalian cells: Epigenetics: advances of non-coding RNAs regulation in mammalian cells. Hereditas (Beijing). 2009;**31**(11):1077-1086

[34] Rutherford ST, Van Kessel JC, Shao Y, et al. AphA and LuxR/HapR reciprocally control quorum sensing in vibrios. Genes & Development. 2011;**25**(4):397-408

[35] Nealson KH, Hastings JW. Bacterial bioluminescence: Its control and ecological significance. Microbiological reviews. 1979;**43**(4):496-518

[36] Papenfort K, Bassler BL. Quorum sensing signal-response systems in Gram-negative bacteria. Nature Reviews. Microbiology. 2016;**14**(9):576-588

[37] Van Kessel JC, Rutherford ST, Shao Y, Utria AF, Bassler BL. Individual and combined roles of the master regulators AphA and LuxR in control of the Vibrio harveyi quorum-sensing regulon. Journal of Bacteriology. 2013;**195**(3):436-443

[38] Shao Y, Feng L, Rutherford ST, Papenfort K, Bassler BL. Functional determinants of the quorum-sensing non-coding RNAs and their roles in target regulation. The EMBO Journal. 2013;**32**(15):2158-2171

[39] Lu R, Osei-Adjei G, Huang X, et al. Role and regulation of the orphan AphA protein of quorum sensing in pathogenic Vibrios. Future Microbiology. 2018;**13**:383-391

[40] Gu D, Liu H, Yang Z, Zhang Y, Wang Q, et al. Chromatin immunoprecipitation sequencing technology reveals global regulatory roles of low-cell-density quorum-sensing regulator AphA in the pathogen V. alginolyticus. Journal of Bacteriology. 2016;**198**(21):2985-2999

[41] Liu H, Liu W, He X, et al. Characterization of a cell density-dependent sRNA, Qrr, and its roles in the regulation of the quorum sensing and metabolism in V. alginolyticus. Applied Microbiology and Biotechnology. 2020;**104**(4):1707-1720

[42] Yang Z, Zhou X, Ma Y, et al. Serine/threonine kinase PpkA coordinates the interplay between T6SS2 activation and quorum sensing in the marine pathogen V. alginolyticus. Environmental Microbiology. 2018;**20**:903-919

[43] Xiating G, Xuetong W, Qiaoqiao M, et al. VqsA, a Novel LysR-Type transcriptional regulator, coordinates quorum sensing (QS) and is controlled by QS to regulate virulence in the pathogen V. alginolyticus. Applied and Environmental Microbiology. 2018;**84**(12):e00444-18

[44] Gao X, Liu Y, Liu H, et al. Identification of the regulon of AphB and its essential roles in LuxR and exotoxin Asp expression in the pathogen V. alginolyticus. Journal of Bacteriology. 2017;**199**(20):e00444-18

[45] Gu D, Guo M, Yang M, et al. A σE-mediated temperature gauge controls a switch from LuxR-mediated virulence gene expression to thermal stress adaptation in V. alginolyticus. PLoS Pathogens. 2016;**12**(6):e1005645

[46] Rui H, Liu Q, Ma Y, et al. Roles of LuxR in regulating extracellular alkaline serine protease A, extracellular polysaccharide and mobility of V. alginolyticus. FEMS Microbiology Letters. 2008;**285**(2):155-162

[47] Liu H, Gu D, Cao X, et al. Characterization of a new quorum sensing regulator luxT and its roles in the extracellular protease production, motility, and virulence in fish pathogen V. alginolyticus. Archives of Microbiology. 2012;**194**(6):439-452

[48] Costerton JW, Geesey GG, Cheng KJ. How bacteria stick. Scientific American. 1978;**238**(1):86-95

[49] Costerton JW, Geesey GG, Cheng KJ, et al. Bacterial biofilms in nature and disease. 1987;**41**:435-464

[50] Flemming HC, Wingender J, Szewzyk U, et al. Biofilms: An emergent form of bacterial life. Nature Reviews. Microbiology. 2016;**14**(9):563-575

[51] Muhsin J, Wisal A, Saadia A, et al. Bacterial biofilm and associated infections. Journal of the Chinese Medical Association. 2018;**81**(1):7-11

[52] Gang Y, Yingxue Q, Wenzheng Z, et al. Study on biofilm formation characteristics of pathogenic V. alginolyticus. Aquatic Science. 2012;**31**(02):73-78

[53] Cvitkovitch DG, Li Y, Ellen RP. Quorum sensing and biofilm formation in Streptococcal infections. The Journal of Clinical Investigation. 2003;**112**(11):1626-1632

[54] Romling U, Balsalobre C. Biofilm infections, their resilience to therapy and innovative treatment strategies. Journal of Internal Medicine. 2012;**272**(6):541-561

[55] Na Zhang, Shun Zhang, Wei Ren, et al. Roles of rpoN in biofilm formation of V. alginolyticus HN08155 at different cell densities. Microbiological Research, 202;**247**:126728

[56] Gu D, Zhang J, Hao Y, et al. Alternative sigma factor RpoX is a part of the RpoE regulon and plays distinct roles in stress responses, motility, biofilm formation, and hemolytic activities in the marine pathogen V. alginolyticus. Applied and Environmental Microbiology. 2019;**85**(14):e00234-19

[57] Petersen FC, Pecharki D, Scheie AA. Biofilm mode of growth of Streptococcus intermedius favored by a competence-stimulating signaling peptide. 2004;**186**:6327-6331

[58] Davies DG, Parsek MR, Pearson JP, et al. The involvement of cell-to-cell signals in the development of a bacterial biofilm. Science (New York, N.Y.). 1998;**280**(5361):295-298

[59] Wen Liang Y, Zhen Yu X, Yan Hua Z, et al. Two (p)ppGpp synthetase genes, relA and spoT, are involved in regulating cell motility, exopolysaccharides production, and biofilm formation of V. alginolyticus. Frontiers in Microbiology. 2022;**13**:858559

[60] Zhang Y, Tan H, Yang S, et al. The role of dctP gene in regulating colonization, adhesion and pathogenicity of V. alginolyticus strain HY9901. Journal of Fish Diseases. 2022;**45**(3):421-434

[61] Chen C, Wang Q-b, Liu Z-H, et al. Characterization of role of the toxR gene in the physiology and pathogenicity of V. alginolyticus. Antonie Van Leeuwenhoek. 2012;**101**:281-288

[62] William HB, Robert AB, Hui W, et al. Oral biofilms: Pathogens, matrix, and polymicrobial interactions

in microenvironments. Trends in Microbiology. 2018;**26**(3):229-242

[63] Hider RC, Kong X. Chemistry and biology of siderophores. Natural Product Reports. 2010;**27**(5):637-657

[64] Schaible UE, Kaufmann SHE. Iron and microbial infection. Nature reviews. Microbiology. 2004;**2**(12):946-953

[65] Crosa JH, Walsh CT. Genetics and assembly line enzymology of siderophore biosynthesis in bacteria. Microbiology and Molecular Biology Reviews: MMBR. 2002;**66**(2):223-249

[66] Challis GL. A widely distributed bacterial pathway for siderophore biosynthesis independent of nonribosomal peptide synthetases. Chembiochem: A European Journal of Chemical Biology. 2005;**6**(4):601-611

[67] Faraldo-Gómez JD, Sansom MSP. Acquisition of siderophores in gram-negative bacteria. Nature Reviews. Molecular Cell Biology. 2003;**4**(2):105-116

[68] Escolar L, Pérez-Martín J, de Lorenzo V. Opening the iron box: Transcriptional metalloregulation by the Fur protein. Journal of Bacteriology. 1999;**181**(20)

[69] CBiosca EG, Fouz B, Alcaide E, et al. Siderophore-mediated iron acquisition mechanisms in V. vulnificus biotype 2. Applied and Environmental Microbiology, 1996,**62**(3):928-935

[70] Christine J, Sebastian S. The role of motility as a virulence factor in bacteria. International Journal of Medical Microbiology. 2002;**291**(8):605-614

[71] Kazmierczak BI, Hendrixson DR. Spatial and numerical regulation of flagellar biosynthesis in polarly flagellated bacteria. Molecular Microbiology. 2013;**88**(4):655-663

[72] Atsumi T, Maekawa Y, Yamada T, et al. Effect of viscosity on swimming by the lateral and polar flagella of V. alginolyticus. Journal of Bacteriology. 1996;**178**(16):5024-5026

[73] Kawagishi I, Nakada M, Nishioka N, Homma M, et al. Cloning of a V. alginolyticus rpoN gene that is required for polar flagellar formation. Journal of Bacteriology. 1997;**179**(21):6851-6854

[74] Yang T, Qiyao W, Qin L, et al. Involvement of LuxS in the regulation of motility and flagella biogenesis in V. alginolyticus. Bioscience, Biotechnology, and Biochemistry. 2008;**72**(4):1063-1071

[75] Shota K, Michio H, Seiji K. Analysis of the GTPase motif of FlhF in the control of the number and location of polar flagella in V. alginolyticus. Biophysics and Physicobiology. 2017;**14**(0):173-181

[76] Correa NE, Peng F, Klose KE. Roles of the regulatory proteins FlhF and FlhG in the V. cholerae flagellar transcription hierarchy. Journal of bacteriology. 2005;**187**(18):6324-6332

[77] Kusumoto A, Kamisaka K, Yakushi T, et al. Regulation of polar flagellar number by the flhF and flhG genes in V. alginolyticus. Journal of biochemistry. 2006;**139**(1):113-121

[78] Balaban M, Hendrixson DR. Polar flagellar biosynthesis and a regulator of flagellar number influence spatial parameters of cell division in Campylobacter jejuni. PLoS pathogens. 2011;7(12):e1002420

[79] Pandza S, Baetens M, Park CH, et al. The G-protein FlhF has a role in polar

flagellar placement and general stress response induction in Pseudomonas putida. Molecular Microbiology. 2000;**36**(2):414-423

[80] Kusumoto A, Shinohara A, Terashima H, et al. Collaboration of FlhF and FlhG to regulate polar-flagella number and localization in V. alginolyticus. Microbiology (Reading, England). 2008;**154**(Pt 5):1390-1399

[81] Zhu S, Nishikino T, Hu B, et al. Molecular architecture of the sheathed polar flagellum in V. alginolyticus. Proceedings of the National Academy of Sciences of the United States of America. 2017;**114**(41):10966-10971

[82] Shinoda S. Protein toxins produced by pathogenic vibrios. Journal of Natural Toxins. 1999;**8**(2):259-269

[83] Sigel SP, Payne SM. Effect of iron limitation on growth, siderophore production, and expression of outer membrane proteins of V. cholerae. Journal of Bacteriology. 1982;**150**(1):148-155

[84] Stoebner JA, Payne SM. Iron-regulated hemolysin production and utilization of heme and hemoglobin by V. cholerae. Infection and Immunity. 1988;**56**(11):2891-2895

[85] Dai JH, Lee YS, Wong HC. Effects of iron limitation on production of a siderophore, outer membrane proteins, and hemolysin and on hydrophobicity, cell adherence, and lethality for mice of Vibrio parahaemolyticus. Infection and Immunity. 1992;**60**(7):2952-2956

[86] Iida H. Hemolysins produced by vibrios. Journal of Toxicology: Toxin Reviews. 1997;**16**(4):215-227

[87] Zhang X, Austin B. Haemolysins in Vibrio species. Journal of Applied Microbiology. 2005;**98**(5):1011-1019

[88] Cai SH, Wu ZH, Jian JC, et al. Cloning and expression of gene encoding the thermostable direct hemolysin from V. alginolyticus strain HY9901, the causative agent of vibriosis of crimson snapper (Lutjanus erythopterus). Journal of Applied Microbiology. 2007;**103**(2):289-296

[89] Liu H, Xiao M, Zuo J, et al. Vanillic acid combats V. alginolyticus by cell membrane damage and biofilm reduction. Journal of Fish Diseases. 2021;**44**(11):1799-1809

[90] Hernández-Robles MF, Álvarez-Contreras AK, Juárez-García P, et al. Virulence factors and antimicrobial resistance in environmental strains of V. alginolyticus. International Microbiology. 2016;**19**(4):191-198

[91] Li L, Meng H, Gu D, et al. Molecular mechanisms of V. parahaemolyticus pathogenesis. Microbiological Research. 2019;**222**:43-51

[92] Morot A, El Fekih S, Bidault A, et al. Virulence of V. harveyi ORM4 towards the European abalone Haliotis tuberculata involves both quorum sensing and a type III secretion system. 2021;**23**:5273-5288

[93] Zhang, T. and M. Yang, Molecular mechanisms of virulence genes expression in V. parahaemolyticus. College of Animal Science and Technology. vol. 60(07). Zhejiang A&F University; 2020. pp. 1345-1357

[94] Cheng H. Function Study of the Virlence Genes acfA and toxR inV. alginolyticus. Guangdong Ocean University; 2014

[95] Quan T, Li W, Yang X. Investigation of the pathogenicity of V. alginolyticus isolated from patients with diarrhea. Chinese Journal of Public Health. 1985;**05**:15-18

[96] Suzuki M, Danilchanka O, Mekalanos JJ, V. cholerae T3SS effector VopE modulates mitochondrial dynamics and innate immune signaling by targeting Miro GTPases. Cell Host Microbe. 2014;**16**(5):581-591

[97] Roehrich AD et al. Steps for shigella gatekeeper protein MxiC function in hierarchical Type III secretion regulation. Journal of Biological Chemistry. 2017;**292**(5):1705-1723

[98] Pang H et al. Acetylome profiling of V. alginolyticus reveals its role in bacterial virulence. Journal of Proteomics. 2020;**211**:103543

[99] Mao F et al. Virulence of V. alginolyticus Accentuates Apoptosis and Immune Rigor in the Oyster Crassostrea hongkongensis. Frontiers in Immunology. 2021;**12**:746017

[100] Wang X, Quinn PJ. Lipopolysaccharide:Biosyntheticpathway and structure modification. Progress in Lipid Research. 2010;**49**(2):97-107

[101] Zhang G, Meredith TC, Kahne D. On the essentiality of lipopolysaccharide to Gram-negative bacteria. Current Opinion in Microbiology. 2013;**16**(6):779-785

[102] Maldonado RF, Sá-Correia I, Valvano MA. Lipopolysaccharide modification in Gram-negative bacteria during chronic infection. FEMS Microbiology Reviews. 2016;**40**(4):480-493

[103] Jian J, Ye J, Wu Z. Influence of lipopolysaccharide fromibrio alginolyticus on immunological function ofepinephelus skaara. Acta Hydrobiologica Sinica. 2004;**01**:103-105

[104] Chen Q, Yan Q, Ma S. Progress on pathogenicity research of V. alginolyticus. Marine Sciences. 2006;**08**:83-89

[105] Xu X et al. A modified silver-staining method for lipopolysaccharides detection. Biotechnology Bulletin. 2009;**03**:95-97

[106] Zhang J et al. Preparation of V. parahaemolyticus lipopolysaccharide and Immunological analysis of the lipopolysaccharide against paralichtys olivaceus. Periodical of Ocean University of China. 2004;**04**:571-576

[107] Smith JA. Brucella Lipopolysaccharide and pathogenicity: The core of the matter. Virulence. 2018;**9**(1):379-382

[108] Zhou Q. Study of Lipid A Structure and Related Genes in V. parahaemolyticus. Southern Yangtze University; 2020

Chapter 6

Radiation-Induced Skin Reactions and Surgical Management Treating Radiation-Induced Ulcers

Hoang Thanh Tuan

Abstract

Radiotherapy (RT) is a cancer treatment that has been widely applied to cancer patients. However, this treatment could induce radiation skin injuries that affect the quality of life of patients. The radiation-induced ulcer is a late-stage complication of radiation burns that could not be self-limited. This chapter summarizes current knowledge relating to RT-induced skin reactions, including epidemiology, pathophysiology, diagnosis, prevention, and management. Additionally, the author also presents the experience of treating RT-induced ulcers by surgical treatments that were shown to give satisfactory results on patients.

Keywords: flap, radiotherapy, radiation treatment, radiation-induced ulcer, single-stage reconstructive surgery

1. Introduction

Radiotherapy (RT) is a measure that delivers radiation to cancer cells that consequently killed these cells. Radiation could be delivered in the form of ionizing particles, photons, or electron beams [1]. Recently, hyperthermia (HT) has been deemed to be a potent radiosensitizer that could enhance the efficacy of radiotherapy in cancer patients [2, 3]. RT-induced skin injuries, or radiation burns, were classified into 4 grades according to Radiation Therapy Oncology Group (RTOG) where the ulceration is included in grade 4 [4].

Although RT brings therapeutic potents to cancer patients, its side effects have been reported in many studies including RT-induced ulcers, which are the most severe situations of radiation burns [4, 5]. The presence of HT, which is often in the combination with RT, in some cases also could increase thermal toxicity [6]. These complications significantly impact patients' quality of life. Thus, a comprehensive understanding of RT-induced ulcers is critical for clinical practices.

This chapter aims to summarize relevant aspects of RT-induced ulcers, including pathophysiology, diagnosis, risks factor of RT-induced skin reactions, epidemiology, prevention, and management of RT-induced skin injuries. The chapter also focuses on the surgical management of RT-induced ulcer, a severe complication of radiation burn.

IntechOpen

2. Pathophysiology

When irradiation performed, the radiation will affect the young cells, makes them to divide rapidly. Therefore, when acting on the skin, radiation causes damage to the germ cells of the skin, hair follicles, sebaceous glands, sweat glands. In the other hand, radiation affects vascular endothelial cells, fibroblasts, etc., thereby causing post-radiotherapy skin lesions. Early-stage common lesions after radiotherapy may be edema, congestion, dry desquamation, moist desquamation, acute ulcers or mild pigmentation disorders. In the late stages, the most common lesions are skin atrophy, sclerosis, loss of skin appendages (hair, sebaceous glands, sweat glands), hyperpigmentation or hypopigmentation, dilated capillaries, vascular lesion, ulcers, necrosis or secondary cancer.

2.1 Mechanism of RT-induced skin reactions

RT-induced skin reactions occurred possibly related to tissue damage and inflammation.

Firstly, radiation could cause DNA breaks due to its ability to release electrons from atoms or molecules. Secondly, it could generate reactive oxygen species resulting in the oxidation of proteins and lipids. Consequently, these effects lead to cell death and the impairment of miotic ability [7]. When a great amount of cell death happened and could not recover, cell death, including basal keratinocytes in the basal layer, would distract the self-renewal ability of the epidermis [8]. As a result, the proliferation of new cells could not completely replace damaged cells resulting in a broken epidermis.

Skin reactions in the epidermis could be followed by inflammation. There is a variety of cytokines and chemokines. They include interleukin IL-1α, IL-1β, TNF-α, TGF-β, IL-6, IL-8, CCL-4, CCL2 [9–11]. The upregulation of these molecules consequently increases the expression of adhesion molecules such as intercellular adhesion molecule-1, vascular cell adhesion molecule, and E-selectin [9, 12, 13]. The transendothelial migration of immune cells from the circulation to damaged areas could be deemed as a hallmark of the inflammatory process.

2.2 Mechanism of RT on wound healing

Normally, the wound healing process undergoes some stages: vasoconstriction and hemostasis (immediately after the lesion), inflammatory reaction (0–3 days), granulation regeneration/reproduction (3 days–3 weeks), repair and recovery (3 weeks–3 years). The wound healing is also influenced by local factors (wound moisture, wound ischemia, bacterial infection) and the systemic ones (congenital pathologies related to collagen deficiency or synthesis, pathologies increasing the risk of bacterial infection and nutrition...).

Influence of radiation on wound healing process [14]:

- Firstly, within the irradiated skin area, the radiation promotes repeated inflammatory reactions, increases the body's inflammatory response, disrupts the cell reproductive regenerative process, causes tissular edema.

- Secondly, the main components involved in the wound healing process are TGFβ, PDGF and FGF. These components are produced by platelets, but radiation suppresses platelet flow to the wound, delaying wound healing.

- Thirdly, radiotherapy directly reduces fibroblasts, the wound elasticity due to decreased collagen production and changed collagen function, thereby delaying the wound healing process.

- Fourthly, radiotherapy causes vascular wall edema, vascular stasis and obstruction, thereby blocking platelets, reducing vascular formation, decreasing cytokines and fibroblasts in wounds, and leads to reduced repair capability of the wound.

According to the study by Hopewell, radiation makes the post-radiotherapy wound healing process more complicated and difficult than other common chronic lesions [15].

3. Diagnosis of radiation-induced skin lesions

Radiation-induced skin lesion is a skin reaction and is also a side effect of radiotherapy in cancer treatment or interventional radiography. There are two types of radiation-induced skin lesion, depending on the time of skin reaction: An acute skin reaction develops hours to weeks after the first exposure to the radiation; The next progression is chronic radiation-induced dermatitis, which may develop months, years or even decades after radiotherapy.

3.1 Manifestations of acute radiation-induced skin lesions

Local changes may occur immediately after irradiation, during the entire course of radiotherapy up to 90 days after radiation. The specific clinical symptoms are as follows [16]:

- Erythema: This is the earliest symptom of acute skin lesions after radiotherapy, initially manifested of light red, which can then turn into bright red or purple red when the dose accumulation increases. Erythema is the result of an inflammatory reaction, characterized by a red blood cell proliferation and dilated capillaries in the dermis.

- Dry skin: Due to the functional reduction of the sebaceous glands, the sweat glands, accompanied by hair brittle and loss.

- Edema: Accompanied by erythema is more edema of irradiated skin. This is the post-irradiated inflammatory reaction of the body that will gradually decrease over time.

- Hyperpigmentation: Skin pigmentation depends on melanin quantity and distribution [17]. Hyperpigmentation is caused by increased activity of melanocytes, which is often accompanied by erythema. This symptom lasts a few months, then may subside [18].

- Dry desquamation: Occurs when the irradiated skin receives a high dose from 3000 cGy, characterized by peeling skin.

- Wet desquamation: Occurs when the epidermis is burned, the underlying surface is wet and edematous, at the dose of above 4000 cGy, common in areas with skin folds. Due to the loss or reduction of the protective function of the epidermis, this expression can form acute ulcers.

- Folliculitis: This is a symptom of the hair follicle infection, manifested by small erythema.

3.2 Manifestations of chronic radiation-induced skin lesions

In order to diagnose chronic radiation-induced skin lesions, it requires an exploitation of medical history and necessary information on radiotherapy including: radiation field, volume, technique, dose, and segmentation, followed by chemotherapy, surgery or other interventions, pre-and post-radiotherapy skin complications. The clinical evaluation is based on consultation and test. The first examination should provide accurate information about the affected areas due to radiotherapy such as lesion area, depth, morphology and color.

In some special cases, when the clinical manifestations are unknown or suspected, a tissue biopsy is required to diagnose: Secondary cancer, angiosarcoma or to distinguish from scleroderma accompanied by radiotherapy. However, biopsies or invasive interventions can worsen radiation-induced fibrosis and prolong ulcerative conditions [18].

3.3 Clinical diagnosis of chronic radiation-induced skin lesions

- Skin atrophy: The most common manifestation of skin atrophy is wrinkles, stronger reactions making skin thin, shiny, scaly. It usually occurs at grade II or III lesions, or may have mild reaction of grade I [19].

- Telangiectasia: occurs in which small blood vessels dilate causing red lines or patterns on the skin, often forms spider veins. This is a common symptom in grade II and III lesions. This symptom may disappear after a short time but may reappear and persist for a long time.

- Radiation-induced fibrosis (RIF): is a condition that subcutaneous tissue after radiotherapy loses connective tissue stability causing the irradiated area to be sclerosis and firmer.

- Dyspigmentation: may appear shortly after irradiation and fade, but may last for months, years or longer. There are two conditions including local hyperpigmentation or hypopigmentation after radiotherapy. According to Ryan et al. and Johansson et al. radiotherapy can cause irreversible damage to pigment cells [19, 20].

- Reduction or loss of skin appendages: Radiation can reduce or destroy all hair follicles, sebaceous glands and sweat glands, cause hair loss, reduce sweat secretion, dry the damaged skin.

- Radiation-induced ulcers: This is a late lesion that can occur anywhere in the body, often in the areas mostly affected by radiation, ulcers tend to grow and spread if not treated promptly.

3.4 Subclinical diagnostic measures of chronic radiation-induced skin lesion

- Sonography: This is a non-invasive diagnostic method, using a probe from 7.5 to 20 MHz that can assess the thickness of the skin layer, as well as the degree of skin sclerosis. A 20 MHz probe can detect epidermis, dermis and subcutaneous fat of about 10 mm deep. A 7.5 MHz probe can investigate further into the radiation-induced aponeurosis, muscle, and fibrosis in subcutaneous tissue as well as deeper ulcers [21].

- Thermography: This method uses infrared camera to determine skin surface and body temperature. Skin surface temperature depends on the subcutaneous vascular system, which indirectly evaluates the subcutaneous vascular distribution. Typically, for patients with necrotic lesions, the surface temperature in that area will be lower than that in the inflammatory area.

- Capillary microscopy: This is a non-invasive method, used for capillary qualification and quantification in hypodermal layers. Finger and toe capillaries are dilated in patients with acute radiation-induced skin lesions, whereas they are smaller or absent in patients with chronic radiation-induced skin lesions. Furthermore, distal subungual hemorrhage can be seen at both acute and chronic stages after radiotherapy.

- Magnetic resonance imaging (MRI): This non-intervention method can assess the signals of the dermis, subcutaneous fat, muscle and bone and tissue morphological changes, then lesions can be identified. For example, a hypersignal on MRI is a result of an increased fluid volume in the tissue, which may be seen in cases of inflammation, edema, or necrosis. If fluid in the tissue decreases, signal on the MRI is decreased, but it is impossible to distinguish whether it is necrosis or inflammation on MRI. MRI images can assess the width and depth of radiation-induced ulcers.

- Bone scintigraphy: Helps assess bone lesion beneath ulcer.

- Histopathology and immunohistochemistry: Helps to diagnose the degree of lesion, structural changes of irradiated skin.

4. Risk factors of radiation-induced ulcers

There are some risk factors associated with the development of radiation dermatitis.

4.1 Radiotherapy-related factors

Higher total dose and higher irradiated volume are possibly related to a higher risk of skin injury [22–24]. Several articles revealed that hypofractionated RT contributed to a lower risk of radiation-induced skin injuries [25, 26]. However, a conflict result was shown as a hyperfractionated regime resulting in preferable outcomes [27]. Besides, intensity-modulated radiotherapy (IMRT) could lead to a reduction of skin reactions compared to 2D radiotherapy [28, 29].

Concurrent chemotherapy (i.g. cetuximab) or concurrent targeted therapy might result in a higher risk of skin injuries induced by RT as well [30–32].

4.2 Patient-related factors

Some regions of the body that are more sensitive to radiation such as the scalp, face, neck, extremities, chest, and abdomen, may be prone to develop skin reactions in patients receiving RT [33]. Patients who are obese (BMI > 30), contract connective tissue diseases, or have skin disorders also have a higher risk of developing radiation burns [34–36]. In addition, there are some genetic polymorphisms that were supposed to increase incidences of radiation dermatitis. They included polymorphisms in ABCA1 and IL12RB2, stefinA3, and S100A8 genes [37, 38].

5. Epidemiology

Skin reactions developed in 95% of patients who received RT [39]. 85% of patients suffered from a moderate to severe skin injury shown in another report [5]. Skin toxicity was mostly observed in patients with head and neck cancer and breast cancer, which occurred in over 50% of this population [40].

6. Prevention of radiation-induced skin reactions

6.1 Modern radiation therapy

To reduce complications on the skin, some modern techniques have been applied and gave promising results, such as IMRT and volumetric-modulated arc therapy (VMAT) [41, 42]. These techniques will deliver radiation doses conformally targeting tumor cells rather than surrounding normal cells, thus, minimizing skin injuries. A hypofractionated regimen, which reduces the period of time to exposure to radiation, also could prevent patients from suffering from skin injuries [43].

6.2 Topical corticosteroids

Topical corticosteroids possess anti-inflammatory properties that inhibit proinflammatory cytokines initiating the early stage of skin reactions [44, 45]. Mometasone furoate, a highly potent corticosteroid, was daily during RT and shown its benefits to prevent skin toxicity compared to placebo [46]. Other topical corticosteroids, namely methylprednisolone and betamethasone, revealed similar effects delaying the onset of RT-induced skin dermatitis [47, 48].

6.3 Skincare

After RT, the protection of the skin from adverse agents should be also paid attention to. These measures include protecting skin from the sun (i.g. by applying sunscreen or wearing a long-sleeve shirt), and daily cleaning irradiated skin with mild soap and water. It should be avoided to use an electric razor, tape, and adhesive on irradiated skin areas to minimize irritation or friction.

7. Managements of radiation-induced ulcers

7.1 Non-surgical managements

Biafine cream, hydrogel or hydrocolloid dressings, human bone marrow mesenchymal stem cells, hyperbaric oxygen, and laser therapy were reported to benefit wound healing [49–53].

Biafine promoted wound healing via the attraction of macrophase, an increase in the ratio of IL-1 to IL-6. IL-1 plays an important role in collagen synthesis and collagenase activation and IL-6 stimulates epidermal growth, thus, enhancing skin healing [54]. Human bone marrow mesenchymal stem cells also inhibit the inflammatory process via downregulation of IL-1β levels, activation of CD80+ macrophages, and upregulation of IL-10. Immunoregulation was considered a mechanism for the healing property of human bone marrow mesenchymal stem cells [55].

Hydrocolloid dressings could form a soft gel when they contact with the wound, therefore, the wound surface could keep its moisture, assisting in the liquefaction and separation of debris [56, 57].

7.2 Surgical management

7.2.1 Management of RT-induced ulcers

Complete excision of lesion both in width and depth is important in treating radiation-induced skin lesions. Many authors agreed to thoroughly treat the lesion before performing covering measures. This helps to eliminate damaged tissue, promote wound healing and reduce the risk of recurrence ulcer as well as the abnormal growth of tissue damaged by radiation. According to research by Wei et al. [58], dividing the cut-off depth is a challenge. Theoretically, the most seriously affected area is within 2 cm below the skin surface. Therefore, the depth of the cut-off is at least 2 cm, but it depends on the anatomical region. Above all, the deep removal into healthy tissues is very important. However, according to the author's experience, no cut-off depth must exceed the muscular layer [58]. In Fujioka's 2012 research and review [59], it is necessary to remove all infiltrated skin area, damaged bones and cartilage to ensure the cleanest wounds before covering. Removing the chest ulcerative lesion in the absence of recurrent cancer, it requires remove the entire non-important structure such as the large skin area, the bone and the cartilage until covering all lesion areas, then performing the defect covering [60].

However, the removal of all lesion is extremely difficult, because the post-radiotherapy lesion usually progresses lately for months and years, not only in width but depth into the structure under the irradiated area, which makes management more complex and difficult.

7.2.2 Plasty techniques of covering post-resection defects

7.2.2.1 Skin grafting

Most authors in the world said that skin grafting was not effective in covering defects for treating radiation-induced ulcers, because radiation damage is an area of atrophied dry tissue with sclerosis and prolonged anemia, inability to form complete granular tissue. According to the research conducted by Strawberry et al. [61], the rate of skin graft failure in his study was nearly 100%. Vu Quang Vinh in his report 2010, also reached the same conclusion, by reporting one case of radiation-induced ulcer, treated with surgical excision and skin graft on average 9 times, grafted skin still was not alive [62].

Some authors used skin grafting method for lesions of radiation with low dose, or after removing thoroughly the lesion, the lesion base/background was well supplied, or used great omentum flap and fascial flap to cover first, then performed the skin grafts [63].

7.2.2.2 Direct closure

Direct closure of the radiation-induced ulcerative lesion usually has low efficiency with high failure rate. Research by Di Meo et al. showed that direct closure is rarely successful with many complications because of poor vascularization at the lesion area [64]. Research by Luce also suggested that direct closure should not be used in treating radiation-induced skin lesions [65].

7.2.2.3 Plasty technique with random flap

Random flap can be used in different forms: sliding flap, rotation flap, rotation-sliding flap, permutation flap.

- Advantages: Softness and elasticity of the flap is compatible with the damaged skin area, the surgery is simple and easy.

- Disadvantages: Limited in area, direction and rotation of the flap. Especially in the case of radiation-induced ulcers, the area surrounding lesions are often infiltrated, extensively sclerotic, not suitable for the use of adjacent flap.

According to Fujioka M.'s report 2012, random flap is not recommended in treating radiation-induced skin lesion, because the peri-ulcerative tissue was contaminated, resulting in poorly supplied blood vessels, delaying the recovery process [59]. In Di Meo et al.' study, they also suggested not choosing random flap because of the high necrotic incidence, so it was preferable to use/select pedicled flaps [64]. According to a study by Strawberry et al. [61], the use of local (random) flaps was also recommended because the peri-ulcerative tissues were often damaged due to radiation, resulting in necrotic flap. However, this kind of flap can still be indicated in case of small area ulcer, early ulcer, low radiation dose, with soft, mobile and well-supplied surroundings.

7.2.2.4 Plasty technique with expander flap

- Advantages: avoid large lesion area during surgery, not affect the function of the donor flap. According to a MacMillan et al.'s study, the peri-lesion skin expansion shall provide tissue with well supplied vessels for the ulceration [66].

- Disadvantages: Non-applicable to lesion areas without hard base. It requires 2 times surgery, risk of bleeding, exposed dermectasia and infection.

With radiation-induced lesions, using the expander flap can still be applied to the narrow soft the areas surrounding lesion.

7.2.2.5 Plasty technique with seamless pedicled flap

Pedicled flaps are taken from a non-irradiated area, which is a good plasty material, the first choice recommended by many authors. In particular, the skin and muscle flap contribute to treating ulcer easier. Marayuma's report in 1986 on plasty coverage of thoracic ulcers with rectus abdominis flap on 16 patients gave good results [67].

- Advantages: After transferring the flap to the new position, the properties of the flap remain unchanged, thus ensuring the esthetics and functionality, without secondary retraction. A great volume of flap can be obtained more easily in cases of post-radiation ulcers [59].

- Disadvantages: The covering ability of the flap is limited because of the length and rotation of the flap. This technique may leave bad scars at flap donor site, difficult direct closure. Sometimes it is not applicable because radiation ulcerative lesions are often accompanied by infiltration and small peri-ulcerative blood vessels.

7.2.2.6 Perforator skin flap

Besides microsurgical and pedicled flaps, perforator flap is also widely used in covering radiation-induced defects. According to Fujioka's study in 2012 [68], knowledge about perforator anatomy helps select covering flap more diversely, adjacent flaps can cover defects instead of the free flap. The most significant advantage of the perforator flap is not to sacrifice any major blood vessels or muscles and minimize the damage to the flap donor site.

However, because radiation-induced lesion is surrounded by scleroris and vascular lesions, the use of perforator flap is only applicable when perforator branch is found far from the lesion area.

7.2.2.7 Free flap transfer with vascular microsurgery

Micro-surgical flap transfer has been extensively used in plastic surgery of radiation-induced ulcer management with high success rate. This technique allows the surgeon to choose the most suitable tissue for the area and the shape of the lesion. The most difficult in using free flap is to find vascular supply on a sclerotic base. Therefore, when using the microsurgical flap to treat radiation-induced ulcers, it requires dissection of a long enough flap pedicle and discovery of the vascular receiver located far away from the irradiated area [69].

In the plasty of radiation-induced ulcer, microsurgical skin flap is often applied to treat head-face-neck ulcers, which is abundant, constant and well-supplied blood vessels. The radiation-induced ulcerative lesions in this area are often complicated, the ulcer can be communicated with the oral cavity or accompanied by bone exposure and geode. Therefore, the plasty material by microscopic flap can meet the requirement of covering both sides (external and oral cavity) with perforator flap separated from one/ the same original vessel or ensure to cover the ulcer by skin flap, and geode formation with microsurgical osteomuscular skin flap.Some consequent reconstructive surgery could be performed to cover defects caused by RT. The uses of full-thickness skin grafts, tissue expanders, random-pattern flaps, perforator flaps or axial-pattern flaps, and free flaps were reported for reconstruction after RT-induced ulcer.

7.2.3 Case illustrations

Deep inferior epigastric perforator (DIEP) free flap and latissimus dorsi muscle flap (LDMF) are commonly used over decades for breast reconstruction. While DIEP is more widely applied because of its advantages, it could be not suitable in some cases because a successful surgery depends on factors consisting of surgeons, equipment, and patients themselves [70–72]. LDMF would be preferable in the case a short duration of sedation is requested. This flap is also more suitable for Asian patients than Caucasian patients because this population requires smaller breast volume. Illustrations of LDMF for breast reconstruction after RT-ulcers are presented in **Figures 1** and **2**. These Asian patients were well-healed after the surgery and no recurrence of ulcer happened.

If deep lesion can affect the blood vessels, pleura, pericardium, it is necessary to carefully examine the lesions on CT or MRI film to see the lesions level related to organizations, thereby taking measures to treat the bottom of the lesions appropriately and safely. Hereby, we presented one female patient born in 1937, who had a left breast ulcer after 30 years of radiotherapy for breast cancer, and ulcer depth reaching the pericardium. Evaluation on CT showed that the boundary between lesions and pericardium is not clear, there is a risk of pericardial lesion during the management of lesions. We have conducted consultation and coordination with the thoracic surgeons during surgery, to ensure the safety for the patient but also need to eliminate all lesions, minimize the risk of cancer or recurrent ulcer after surgery. The patient was treated with maximum width and depth of lesion, using large back muscle skin flap to cover the defect. Skin flap was good after surgery. The incision healed in the cycle 1. No ulcer recurrence occurred after 3 year (**Figure 3**).

Free flaps are also common options due to their good vascularization and rapid healing. **Figure 4** describes a case of a 44-year-old male patient who had an ulcer on his neck after RT. A free flap was used in this patient after the excision of the ulcer. Three months postoperatively, a favorable result was observed.

Superior gluteal artery perforator flaps could be useful in the cases of RT-ulcer on the buttock region. The reconstructive surgery gave a favorable result in a 44-year-old male patient after the excision of RT-induced ulcer on his button (**Figure 5**).

In addition, in the case to avoid intensive surgery and/or to minimize defects on the donor site, a tissue expander or random-pattern flap could be appropriate

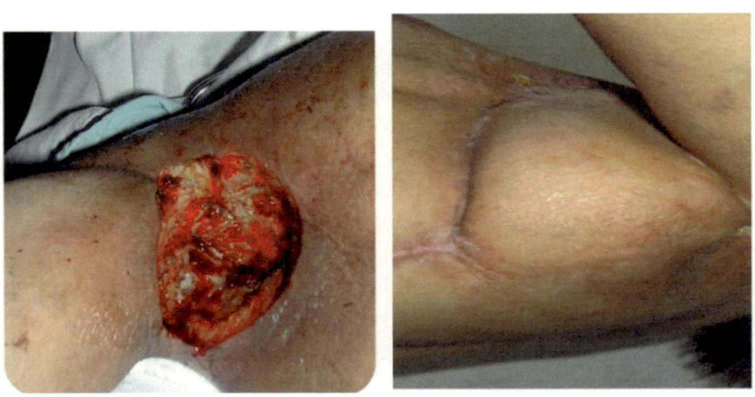

Figure 1.
A 59-year-old female patient with a ulcer at her axilla after RT (left). The wound was debrided and then covered by LDMF (right).

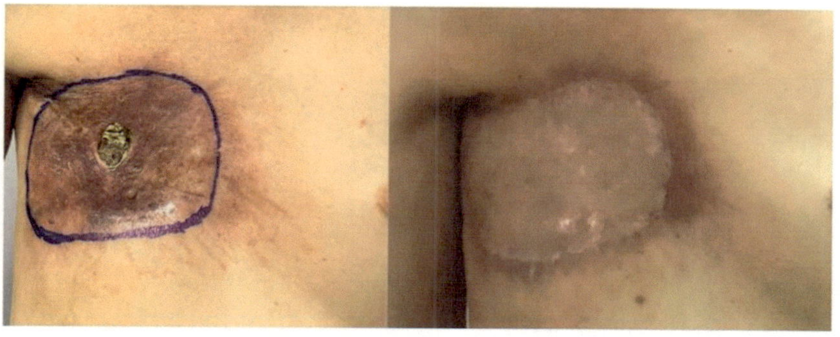

Figure 2.
A 55-year-old patient with a ulcer on her chest along with wide infiltrated and fibrotic areas (left). She underwent debridement followed by a reconstruction with LDMF (right).

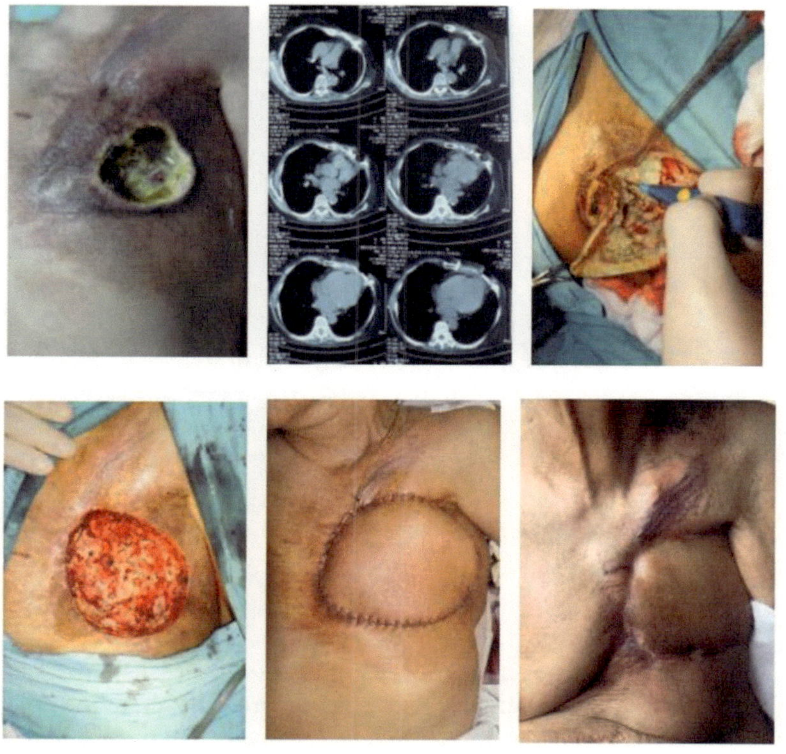

Figure 3.
Illustration of a RT-induced ulcer case with exposed pericardium. (Above, lef) Before the surgery. (Above, middle) MRI film showed ulcer deep to the pericardium. (Above, right) Lesion removal. (Below, left) After cutting the whole lesion. (Below, middle) 1 week after surgery. (Below, right) 3 years after the surgery.

choices. The expanded flaps have benefits in terms of good blood supply to tissues of RT-induced wounds, minor complications, and satisfactory esthetic results. Necrotic areas and total infiltrated areas should be entirely removed in the cases of first-degree and second-degree ulcers. In the meanwhile, partial excision would be more appropriate for other ulcers because of a dense vessel system or ribs underneath the wound. Generally, if the base of ulcers could not be completely monitored, drainage should be placed for a long time.

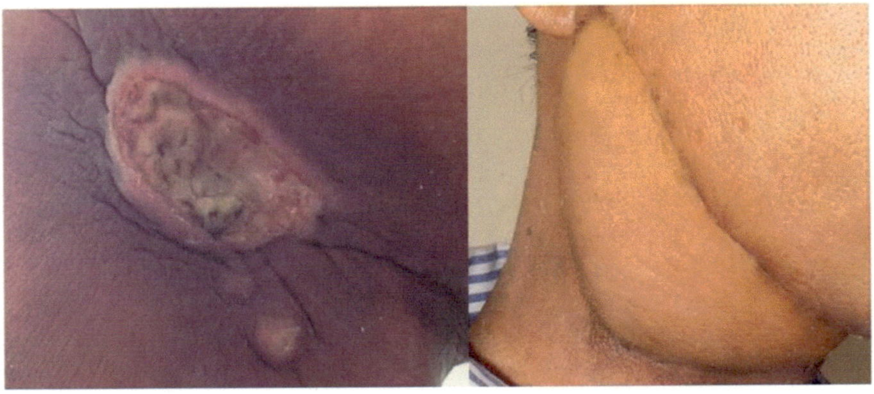

Figure 4.
The RT-ulcer appeared on the neck of patient (A). A favorable result was seen after 3 months.

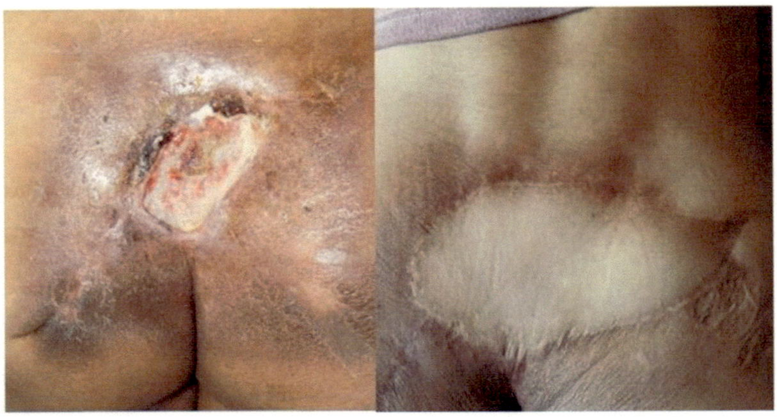

Figure 5.
RT-ulcer on button of a male patient. (Left) Before the surgery. (Right) 3 months after the surgery.

8. Conclusions

Radiation burn is a common and severe complication after RT that affected a majority of patients. This chapter provided some general data about the epidemiology, diagnosis, pathophysiology, prevention, and management of RT-induced skin reactions. In addition, the RT-induced ulcer, which is a severe form of radiation burn, could be effectively treated by excision and reconstructive surgery with varied flaps.

Conflict of interest

The author declares no conflict of interest.

Author details

Hoang Thanh Tuan
National Burns Hospital, Hanoi, Vietnam

*Address all correspondence to: tuanht.vb@gmail.com

References

[1] Gazda MJ, Coia LRJC. Principles of radiation therapy. Cancer Network. 2001;**26**:9-19

[2] Kaur P, Hurwitz MD, Krishnan S, Asea AJC. Combined hyperthermia and radiotherapy for the treatment of cancer. Cancers. 2011;**3**(4):3799-3823

[3] Peeken JC, Vaupel P, Combs SE. Integrating hyperthermia into modern radiation oncology: What evidence is necessary?. Frontiers in oncology. 2017;**7**:132

[4] Cox JDJ. Toxicity criteria of the radiation therapy oncology group (RTOG) and the European organization for research and treatment of cancer (EORTC). International Journal of Radiation Oncology, Biology, Physics. 1995;**31**:1341-1346

[5] Bolderston A, Lloyd NS, Wong RK, Holden L, Robb-Blenderman LJS. The prevention and management of acute skin reactions related to radiation therapy: A systematic review and practice guideline. Supportive Care in Cancer. 2006;**14**(8):802-817

[6] Bakker A, van der Zee J, van Tienhoven G, Kok HP, Rasch CR, Crezee HJI. Temperature and thermal dose during radiotherapy and hyperthermia for recurrent breast cancer are related to clinical outcome and thermal toxicity: A systematic review. International Journal of Hyperthermia. 2019;**36**(1):1023-1038

[7] Borrego-Soto G, Ortiz-López R, Rojas-Martínez AJG. Ionizing radiation-induced DNA injury and damage detection in patients with breast cancer. Genetics and molecular biology. 2015;**38**:420-432

[8] Harper JL, Franklin LE, Jenrette JM, Aguero EGJS. Skin toxicity during breast irradiation: Pathophysiology and management. Southern medical journal. 2004;**97**(10):989-994

[9] Holler V, Buard V, Gaugler M-H, Guipaud O, Baudelin C, Sache A, et al. Pravastatin limits radiation-induced vascular dysfunction in the skin. Journal of investigative dermatology. 2009;**129**(5):1280-1291

[10] Okunieff P, Xu J, Hu D, Liu W, Zhang L, Morrow G, et al. Curcumin protects against radiation-induced acute and chronic cutaneous toxicity in mice and decreases mRNA expression of inflammatory and fibrogenic cytokines. International Journal of Radiation Oncology* Biology* Physics. 2006;**65**(3):890-898

[11] Xiao Z, Su Y, Yang S, Yin L, Wang W, Yi Y, et al. Protective effect of esculentoside A on radiation-induced dermatitis and fibrosis. International Journal of Radiation Oncology* Biology* Physics. 2006;**65**(3):882-889

[12] Müller K, Meineke VJE. Radiation-induced alterations in cytokine production by skin cells. Experimental hematology. 2007;**35**(4):96-104

[13] Yuan H, Goetz DJ, Gaber MW, Issekutz AC, Merchant TE, MFJ K. Radiation-induced up-regulation of adhesion molecules in brain microvasculature and their modulation by dexamethasone. Radiation research. 2005;**163**(5):544-551

[14] Bentzen SMJNRC. Preventing or reducing late side effects of radiation therapy: Radiobiology meets molecular pathology. Nature Reviews Cancer. 2006;**6**(9):702-713

[15] Hopewell JW. The skin: Its structure and response to ionizing radiation.

International journal of radiation biology. 1990;**57**(4):751-773

[16] Arron S. Anatomy of the skin and pathophysiology of radiation dermatitis. In: Skin care in radiation oncology. Cham, Switzerland: Springer; 2016. pp. 9-14

[17] Nielsen KP, Zhao L, Stamnes JJ, Stamnes K, Moan J. The importance of the depth distribution of melanin in skin for DNA protection and other photobiological processes. Journal of Photochemistry and Photobiology. B: Biology. 2006;**82**(3):194-198

[18] Fowble B, Yom SS, Yuen F. Types of radiation-related skin reactions. In: Skin Care in Radiation Oncology. Cham, Switzerland: Springer; 2016. pp. 15-29

[19] Spałek M. Chronic radiation-induced dermatitis: Challenges and solutions. Clinical, cosmetic and investigational dermatology. 2016;**9**:473

[20] Johansson S, Svensson H, Denekamp J. Dose response and latency for radiation-induced fibrosis, edema, and neuropathy in breast cancer patients. International Journal of Radiation Oncology* Biology* Physics. 2002;**52**(5):1207-1219

[21] Ralf UP, Petra G. Management of cutaneous radiation injuries: Diagnostic and therapeutic principles of the cutaneous radiation syndrome. Military medicine. 2002;**167**:110-112

[22] Cuttino LW, Heffernan J, Vera R, Rosu M, Ramakrishnan VR, Arthur DW. Association between maximal skin dose and breast brachytherapy outcome: A proposal for more rigorous dosimetric constraints. International Journal of Radiation Oncology* Biology* Physics. 2011;**81**(3):e173-e177

[23] Geara FB, Komaki R, Tucker SL, Travis EL, Cox JDJ. Factors influencing the development of lung fibrosis after chemoradiation for small cell carcinoma of the lung: Evidence for inherent interindividual variation. International Journal of Radiation Oncology* Biology* Physics. 1998;**41**(2):279-286

[24] Collette S, Collette L, Budiharto T, Horiot JC, Poortmans PM, Struikmans H, et al. Predictors of the risk of fibrosis at 10 years after breast conserving therapy for early breast cancer–A study based on the EORTC trial 22881-10882 'boost versus no boost'. European Journal of Cancer. 2008;**44**(17):2587-2599

[25] Jagsi R, Griffith KA, Boike TP, Walker E, Nurushev T, Grills IS, et al. Differences in the acute toxic effects of breast radiotherapy by fractionation schedule: Comparative analysis of physician-assessed and patient-reported outcomes in a large multicenter cohort. JAMA oncology. 2015;**1**(7):918-930

[26] James M, Lehman M, Hider PN, Jeffery M, Hickey BE, Francis DP. Fraction size in radiation therapy for breast conservation in early breast cancer. Cochrane Database of Systematic Reviews. 2016;**7**

[27] Saunders M, Dische S, Barrett A, Harvey A, Griffiths G, Parmar M. Continuous, hyperfractionated, accelerated radiotherapy (CHART) versus conventional radiotherapy in non-small cell lung cancer: Mature data from the randomised multicentre trial. Radiotherapy and Oncology. 1999;**52**(2):137-148

[28] Barnett GC, Wilkinson JS, Moody AM, Wilson CB, Twyman N, Wishart GC, et al. Randomized controlled trial of forward-planned intensity modulated radiotherapy for early breast cancer: Interim results at

2 years. International Journal of Radiation Oncology* Biology* Physics. 2012;**82**(2):715-723

[29] Donovan E, Bleakley N, Denholm E, Evans P, Gothard L, Hanson J, et al. Randomised trial of standard 2D radiotherapy (RT) versus intensity modulated radiotherapy (IMRT) in patients prescribed breast radiotherapy. Radiotherapy and Oncology. 2007;**82**(3):254-264

[30] Satzger I, Degen A, Asper H, Kapp A, Hauschild A, Gutzmer RJJ. Serious skin toxicity with the combination of BRAF inhibitors and radiotherapy. Journal of Clinical Oncology: Official Journal of the American Society of Clinical Oncology. 2013;**31**(13):e220-e222

[31] Anker CJ, Grossmann KF, Atkins MB, Suneja G, Tarhini AA, Kirkwood JM. Avoiding severe toxicity from combined BRAF inhibitor and radiation treatment: Consensus guidelines from the Eastern Cooperative Oncology Group (ECOG). International Journal of Radiation Oncology* Biology* Physics. 2016;**95**(2):632-646

[32] Toledano A, Garaud P, Serin D, Fourquet A, Bosset J-F, Breteau N, et al. Concurrent administration of adjuvant chemotherapy and radiotherapy after breast-conserving surgery enhances late toxicities: Long-term results of the ARCOSEIN multicenter randomized study. International Journal of Radiation Oncology* Biology* Physics. 2006;**65**(2):324-332

[33] Brown KR, Rzucidlo EJ. Acute and chronic radiation injury. Journal of vascular surgery. 2011;**53**(1):15S-21S

[34] Thomas A, Keller A, Menoux I, Brahimi Y, Vigneron C, Le Fèvre C, et al. Prognostic factors of acute radiodermatitis in breast cancer after adjuvant radiotherapy treated with RT3D or IMRT. Cancer Radiotherapie: Journal de la Societe Francaise de Radiotherapie Oncologique. 2022;**26**(5):684-691

[35] Hölscher T, Bentzen SM, Baumann MJR. Influence of connective tissue diseases on the expression of radiation side effects: A systematic review. Radiotherapy and Oncology. 2006;**78**(2):123-130

[36] Hymes SR, Strom EA, Fife C. Radiation dermatitis: Clinical presentation, pathophysiology, and treatment 2006. Journal of the American Academy of Dermatology. 2006;**54**(1):28-46

[37] Isomura M, Oya N, Tachiiri S, Kaneyasu Y, Nishimura Y, Akimoto T, et al. IL12RB2 and ABCA1 genes are associated with susceptibility to radiation dermatitis. Clinical Cancer Research. 2008;**14**(20):6683-6689

[38] Kuptsova N, Chang-Claude J, Kropp S, Helmbold I, Schmezer P, von Fournier D, et al. Genetic predictors of long-term toxicities after radiation therapy for breast cancer. International Journal of Cancer. 2008;**122**(6):1333-1339

[39] Ryan JLJ. Ionizing radiation: The good, the bad, and the ugly. Journal of Investigative Dermatology. 2012;**132**(3):985-993

[40] Chan RJ, Mann J, Tripcony L, Keller J, Cheuk R, Blades R, et al. Natural oil-based emulsion containing allantoin versus aqueous cream for managing radiation-induced skin reactions in patients with cancer: A phase 3, double-blind, randomized, controlled trial. British Journal of School Nursing. 1999;**8**(17):1134-1140

[41] Teoh M, Clark C, Wood K, Whitaker S, Nisbet A. Volumetric

modulated arc therapy: A review of current literature and clinical use in practice. The British journal of Radiology. 2011;**84**(1007):967-996

[42] Pignol J-P, Olivotto I, Rakovitch E, Gardner S, Sixel K, Beckham W, et al. A multicenter randomized trial of breast intensity-modulated radiation therapy to reduce acute radiation dermatitis. Journal of Clinical Oncology. 2008;**26**(13):2085-2092

[43] Shaitelman SF, Schlembach PJ, Arzu I, Ballo M, Bloom ES, Buchholz D, et al. Acute and short-term toxic effects of conventionally fractionated vs hypofractionated whole-breast irradiation: A randomized clinical trial. JAMA Oncology. 2015;**1**(7):931-941

[44] Beetz A, Oppel T, Lu-Hesselmann J, Peter R, Messer G, Kind PJR. Induction of interleukin-6 by ionizing radiation in a human epithelial cell line. Modulation by corticosteroids. Radioprotection. 1997;**32**:319-320

[45] Meghrajani CF, Co HCS, Ang-Tiu CMU, Roa FCJ. Topical corticosteroid therapy for the prevention of acute radiation dermatitis: A systematic review of randomized controlled trials. Expert Review of Clinical Pharmacology. 2013;**6**(6):641-649

[46] Miller RC, Schwartz DJ, Sloan JA, Griffin PC, Deming RL, Anders JC, et al. Mometasone furoate effect on acute skin toxicity in breast cancer patients receiving radiotherapy: a phase III double-blind, randomized trial from the North Central Cancer Treatment Group N06C4. International Journal of Radiation Oncology* Biology* Physics. 2011;**79**(5):1460-1466

[47] Schmuth M, Wimmer M, Hofer S, Sztankay A, Weinlich G, Linder D, et al. Topical corticosteroid therapy for acute radiation dermatitis: A prospective, randomized, double-blind study. British Journal of Dermatology. 2002;**146**(6):983-991

[48] Omidvari S, Saboori H, Mohammadianpanah M, Mosalaei A, Ahmadloo N, Mosleh-Shirazi MA, et al. Topical betamethasone for prevention of radiation dermatitis. Indian Journal of Dermatology, Venereology & Leprology. 2007;**73**(3):209

[49] Krausz AE, Adler BL, Landriscina A, Rosen JM, Musaev T, Nosanchuk JD, et al. Biafine topical emulsion accelerates excisional and burn wound healing in mice. Archives of dermatological research. 2015;**307**(7):583-594

[50] Wasiak J, Cleland H, Campbell F, Spinks AJC. Dressings for superficial and partial thickness burns. Cochrane Database of Systematic Reviews. 2013, Issue 3. Article: CD002106

[51] Agay D, Scherthan H, Forcheron F, Grenier N, Hérodin F, Meineke V, et al. Multipotent mesenchymal stem cell grafting to treat cutaneous radiation syndrome: Development of a new minipig model. Experimental Hematology. 2010;**38**(10):945-956

[52] Yildiz S, Cimsit M, Ilgezdi S, Uzun G, Gumus T, Qyrdedi T, et al. Hyperbaric oxygen therapy used to treat radiation injury: Two case reports. Ostomy/wound Management. 2006;**52**(5):14-16

[53] Schindl A, Schindl M, Pernerstorfer-Schön H, Mossbacher U, Schindl LJP. Low intensity laser irradiation in the treatment of recalcitrant radiation ulcers in patients with breast cancer–long-term results of 3 cases. Photodermatology, photoimmunology & photomedicine. 2000;**16**(1):34-37

[54] Coulomb B, Friteau L, Dubertret L. Biafine applied on human epidermal wounds is chemotactic for macrophages and increases the IL1/IL6 ratio. Skin Pharmacology and Physiology. 1997;**10**(5-6):281-287

[55] Horton JA, Hudak KE, Chung EJ, White AO, Scroggins BT, Burkeen JF, et al. Mesenchymal stem cells inhibit cutaneous radiation-induced fibrosis by suppressing chronic inflammation. Stem cells. 2013;**31**(10):2231-2241

[56] Margolin SG, Breneman JC, Denman DL, LaChapelle P, Weckbach L, Aron BS. Erratum: Management of radiation-induced moist skin desquamation using hydrocolloid dressing. Cancer Nursing. 1990;**13**(4):267

[57] Fisher J, Scott C, Stevens R, Marconi B, Champion L, Freedman GM, et al. Randomized phase III study comparing Best Supportive Care to Biafine as a prophylactic agent for radiation-induced skin toxicity for women undergoing breast irradiation: Radiation Therapy Oncology Group (RTOG) 97-13. International Journal of Radiation Oncology* Biology* Physics. 2000;**48**(5):1307-1310

[58] Wei KC, Yang KC, Chen LW, Liu WC, Chen WC, Chiou WY, et al. Management of fluoroscopy-induced radiation ulcer: One-stage radical excision and immediate reconstruction. Scientific reports. 2016;**6**(1):1-6

[59] Fujioka M. Surgical reconstruction of radiation injuries. Advances in wound care. 2014;**3**(1):25-37

[60] Arnold PG, Pairolero PC. Reconstruction of the radiation-damaged chest wall. Surgical Clinics of North America. 1989;**69**(5):1081-1089

[61] Strawberry CW, Jacobs JS, McCraw JB. Reconstruction for cervical irradiation ulcers with myocutaneous flaps. Head & Neck Surgery. 1984;**6**(4):836-841

[62] Vu QV. Management of radiation ulcers by surgical treatment. Journal of Wound Technology. 2010:65-66

[63] van Geel AN, Contant CM, Wiggers T. Full thickness resection of radiation-induced ulcers of the chest wall: reconstruction with absorbable implants, pedicled omentoplasty, and split skin graft. The European journal of surgery. 1998;**164**(4):305-307

[64] Di Meo L, Jones BM. Surgical treatment of radiation-induced scalp lesions. British journal of plastic surgery. 1984;**37**(3):373-378

[65] Luce EA. The irradiated wound. The Surgical Clinics of North America. 1984;**64**(4):821-829

[66] MacMillan RW, Arias JD, Stayman III JW. Management of radiation necrosis of the chest wall following mastectomy: a new treatment option. Plastic and reconstructive surgery. 1986;**77**(5):832-835

[67] Maruyama Y, Onishi K, Iwahira Y. Reconstructing chest walls with vertical abdominal fasciocutaneous flaps. Scandinavian Journal of Plastic and Reconstructive Surgery. 1986;**20**(1):79-83

[68] Fujioka M, Hayashida K, Murakami C. Resurfacing patella using pedicled soleus perforator flap. Techniques in Knee Surgery. 2012;**11**(3):147-150

[69] Hoffman GR, Islam S, Eisenberg RL. Microvascular reconstruction of the mouth, face and jaws. Oromandibular reconstruction–free fibula

flap. Australian Dental Journal. 2012;**57**(3):379-387

[70] Hunsinger V, Hivelin M, Derder M, Klein D, Velten M, Lantieri L. Long-term follow-up of quality of life following DIEP flap breast reconstruction. Plastic and Reconstructive Surgery. 2016;**137**(5):1361-1371

[71] Hauck T, Horch RE, Schmitz M, Arkudas A. Secondary breast reconstruction after mastectomy using the DIEP flap. Surgical Oncology. 2018;**27**(3):513

[72] Wade RG, Razzano S, Sassoon EM, Haywood RM, Ali RS, Figus A. Complications in DIEP flap breast reconstruction after mastectomy for breast cancer: a prospective cohort study comparing unilateral versus bilateral reconstructions. Annals of surgical oncology. 2017;**24**(6):1465-1474

Chapter 7

Thermal Protective Performance of Turnout Gear at High Flux Environment

Rumeel Ahmad Bhutta and Sengkwan Choi

Abstract

Thermal protective performance (TPP) tests are conducted at a heat flux of 84 kW/m^2 to evaluate a firefighter's turnout gear performance. The test criterion used is based on a study conducted by Behnke in 1984. However, an average heat flux of 200 kW/m^2 has been documented in the literature over the past decade. Henceforth, experiments are conducted on the turnout gear at a higher heat flux level of 126 kW/m^2, which represents a typical heat flux during the initial phase of a fully developed fire. The analytical analysis provides insights into air gaps, the effect of smoke layers on radiative attenuation and the thermal decomposition of the fabric layers. Numerical techniques were employed to introduce a survival curve to effectively gauge the degree of spatial burn at variable levels of heat fluxes, moisture effects and superficial burns. The sustainability of high resistance fabrics in terms of toxicity of flame retardants and recycling of these textiles have been discussed. Bio-composites as flame retardants are being introduced to replace traditional flame-retardant chemicals.

Keywords: firefighter, high heat flux, survival curve, thermal protective clothing, turnout gear

1. Introduction

Turnout gear is worn to safeguard individuals employed in hazardous fields like firefighting, high-speed sports, the oil and gas industry and the military. The protective gear can be either thermal protective clothing for firefighting, chemical resistant clothing for the oil and gas industry or puncture- and cut-resilient clothing for the military [1]. Thermal protective clothing is crucial for firefighters because fire is a common occurrence and poses a significant threat to people's safety. Firefighter protective clothing can be divided into two types: station wear, which is a single-layer garment worn while at the fire station, and turnout gear, which is a multiple-layer garment worn while responding to a fire incident [2]. The turnout gear is a combination of three fabric layers: an outer shell (OS), a moisture barrier (MB) and a thermal liner (TL).

The outer shell is the primary layer in a multi-layered clothing system and is part of a family of fabrics that are naturally resistant to fire [3, 4]. It has a highly organized structure of aromatic groups attached to a backbone chain, which prevents it from breaking down into smaller molecules and producing less smoke when exposed to fire [5, 6]. When this aramid fabric group is combined with other fire-resistant materials using lamination, coating or bonding, it creates a moisture barrier. This porosity of the membrane is a determining factor in moisture control, that is, it is permeable to sweat vapor and acts as a barrier for water droplets. To make a thermal liner, a batting fabric made from fire-resistant fibers is sewn or quilted onto a face fabric, which is also made using fire-resistant fibers. Its main function is to reduce heat dissipation, provide comfort and release metabolic heat away from the wearer's body.

The maximum evaluation criterion for thermal protective clothing was proposed by Behnke [7]. He exposed swatches of the protective fabric made of Nomex®IIIA to several incident fluxes. The amount of incident flux that replicated the appearance from damaged clothing was estimated to be 84 kW/m^2($\approx$2 cal/cm^2s) for 8 seconds of exposure. This estimated value was proposed to be a representation of flashover.

The conditions of a fire, whether it's inside a building or in a forest, can vary from one incident to another due to the unpredictable nature of the materials that are burning [8]. That is why firefighters' protective clothing is designed to be effective under a range of heat levels that are representative of several types of fires, including flashovers, backdrafts, fully developed fires, and forest fires. These garments are classified into routine, hazardous and emergency categories [9, 10]. Recent experiments [11–19] reported an average of 200 kW/m^2 heat flux under extreme conditions in buildings and other enclosed spaces. These are higher levels of fire severity than previously measured. Henceforth, a new upper limit of 126 kW/m^2 is recommended, and the performance of turnout gear is tested at this level.

It corelates with the building data collected by the end of the past decade which emphasize modern construction trends in the housing sector [20, 21]. According to this data, the home area has increased by approximately 232.3 m^2 in 2008, as compared to 144 m^2 in 1973. The 26% of homes built in 2008 were bigger than 278.7 m^2; additionally, a growth of 56% in the construction of 2-storey homes (1-level above ground floor, US standard) was reported. Also, the current housing incorporates taller ceilings of 4.3–6.1 m, than the traditional 2.4 m. All these factors contribute to increased area and volume. As a result, the smoke spread during a fire incident remains above the ongoing fire; hence, more oxygen is available, causing the fire to grow rapidly and violently. This fire spread is also linked to the decorations and contents in the accommodation that have transitioned from natural to synthetic materials, such as cotton being replaced by polyurethane foam [22].

The effectiveness of a multi-layered protective garment can be evaluated using either a full-scale manikin test or a laboratory bench-scale test using the TPP rating system [23–25]. A full-scale manikin test assesses the performance of the entire garment against a convective/radiative thermal load, while a bench-scale test is performed on small patches of the garment. To capture thermal load on the skin, full-scale manikin testing facilities have been developed using a network of over 100 sensors distributed across the manikin's surface [26–30]. However, due to the high cost of full-scale tests, bench-scale tests are preferred as they are more affordable and can still replicate real-world room fires. Standards for bench-scale tests have been developed for diverse types of thermal loads, such as convective, radiant or a mix of both. The assessment criteria such as ISO 9151 [31], ISO 6942 [32], ASTM F2702 [33], ISO 17492 [24], ASTM F2703 [34] and NFPA 1971 [35] vary depending on the heat source and are representative of several types of fire incidents. The data from these experiments are then input into analytical models to predict skin burns.

1.1 Skin burns

The skin layers of interest in burn degree evaluation are the epidermis, dermis and subcutaneous. The second layer, dermis, is of the most significance as its temperature profile corelates to second-degree burns. The human body maintains a skin temperature of 37°C during daily activities. Pain is induced when the body temperature increases by 8°C, which occurs at a temperature of 44°C. A first-degree (superficial) burn occurs at 48°C, and a second-degree burn occurs with continued exposure to heat at 55°C. At 72°C, the skin tissues cannot sustain thermal equilibrium and are destroyed. Two widely accepted criteria are applied to assess this damage, Stoll's and Henrique's.

Stoll's criterion is applied to evaluate protection against second-degree burns [36]. It involves recording temperature data from a benchtop test, and the intersection of the experimental curve with Stoll's documented experimental curve predicts tolerance time. This criterion assumes a rectangular heat pulse, and its validity depends on this assumption.

In contrast, Henrique's is based on a chemical rate process and uses temperature and time to determine skin damage [37]. Skin-simulant sensors are used in modern thermal manikin experiments to predict third-degree burns using Henrique's burn integral, Ω, as shown in Eq. 1. The values of physical constant have been presented in **Table 1**. While Stoll's criterion is easy to use, Henrique integral has shown more accurate predictions for incident heat flux range not covered experimentally by Stoll. Henceforth, it is a preferred choice when assessing superficial burns at heat fluxes above 41 kW/m^2.

$$\Omega = \int_0^t P\exp\left(-\frac{\Delta E}{RT}\right) dt \qquad (1)$$

Ω, Henrique integral, second-degree burn occurs when Ω is unity
ΔE, the activation energy (J/mol)
P, a pre-exponential factor
T, time-dependent absolute temperature of the basal layer.

Constant	Basel layer	Dermal base	Limit
Ω	≤ 0.50, no burn	$\cong 1$, third-degree	—
	$= 0.53$, first-degree		
	$\cong 1.00$, second-degree		
P (1/second)	2.185×10^{124}	4.32×10^{64}	$44 \leq T \leq 50^{\circ}C$
	1.823×10^{51}	9.39×10^{104}	$T \geq 50^{\circ}C$
$\frac{\Delta E}{R}$(K)	93,534.9	50,000	$44 \leq T \leq 50^{\circ}C$
	39,109.8	80,000	$T \geq 50^{\circ}C$

Table 1.
Henrique burn model physical constant values [8, 38].

2. Experimental methodology

To conduct novel tests on the thermal protective garment subjected to a fire load of 126 kW/m^2, a purpose-built experimental apparatus was designed by cooperation between the Korean Conformity Laboratories (KCL) and Ulster University (UU), as shown in **Figure 1**. It comprises a radiant panel, a specimen assembly and a trolley. Two-layered halogen quartz tubes can output a consistent radiant flux of 126 kW/m^2 for more than 60 seconds. More details on the development, configuration and limitations of the test apparatus can be found in the preliminary study of KCL [39].

The experimental setup consists of an outer shell (OS), a moisture barrier (MB), a thermal liner (TL) and a substrate. The addition of a substrate represents closed-back configuration with variations in the air gap between the skin and the innermost layer [40, 41]. The temperature measurement at the back surface of the thermal liner is vital. Therefore, four type-K thermocouples were prepared to record the thermal liner back surface temperature. Constant contact is needed between the thermocouples and thermal liner back surface, for which sewing of the thermocouple was first implemented, as suggested by the National Institute of Standard and Technology (NIST) [42]. However, it was difficult to keep the bead in contact with fabric; plus, sewing made it demanding to retain the stripped wire away from the fabric surface. As four thermocouples are required to be placed in proper contact with the back surface, sewing proved to be impractical. Additionally, the application of heat-resistant tape is not recommended [42]. To overcome this, a new mechanism was developed based on pressure contact.

Thermocouple beads were soldered to a copper sheet of circular cut with a thickness of 0.35 mm. Thermocouple wires ran across the slits on a rod made of high thermal-resistant plastic. It was then put through circular holes in the substrate. The distance between the copper sheet and the circular rod was kept to greater than 6 mm to ensure proper air circulation. In this manner, four probes were prepared and attached at four distinct points of the fabric back surface. This method of pressure contact can record the spatial variations of the temperature, and it has been validated [43].

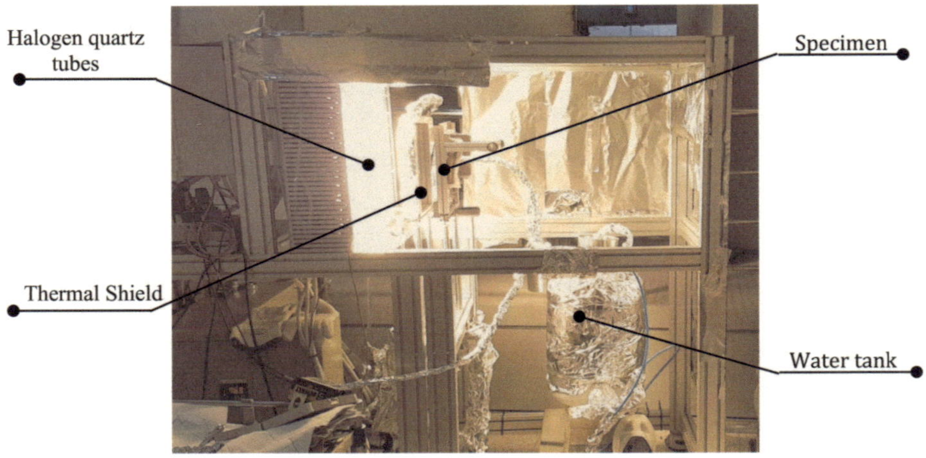

Figure 1.
Bench-scale apparatus.

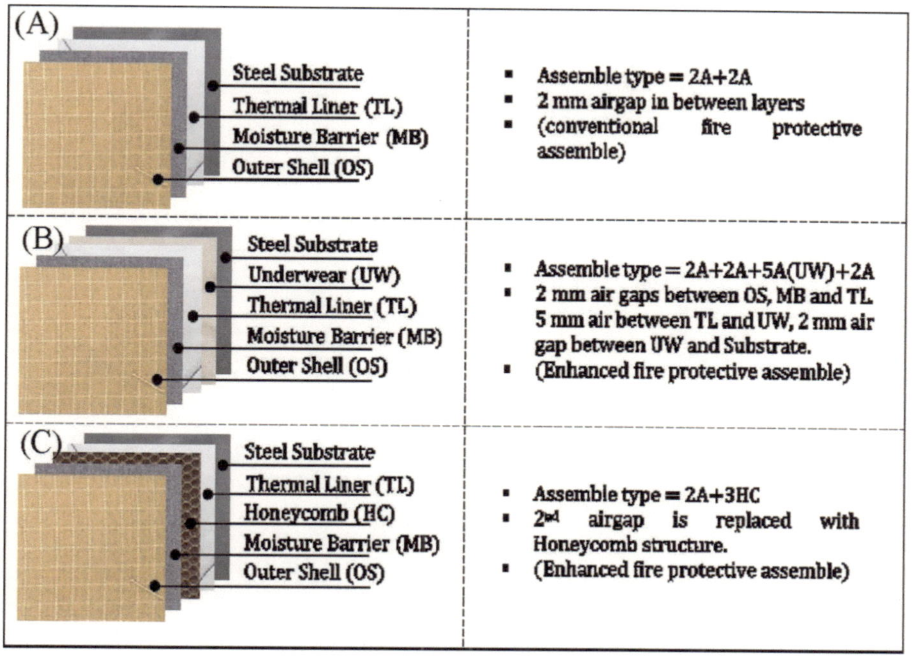

Figure 2.
Turnout gear layup for experimental studies.

Three types of fabric configurations, Type A, B and C as described in **Figure 2**, were examined at two different exposure levels of 84 and 126 kW/m^2, representative of flashover and post-flashover. Specimens were exposed to the incident radiant flux for three different exposure times, of 10, 20 and 25 seconds. Type-A configuration is of a conventional layup. It is commercially available in the market and, therefore, is treated as a benchmark to access the performance of Type B and C. A 2 mm (2A) air spacing is ensured between the fabric layers and 6.5 mm between TL and substrate as per research standards [29, 41, 42, 44].

2.1 Turnout gear characteristics

The functional characteristics of each fabric layer in the turnout gear are distinctive. The OS resists heat; protects the wearer from chemical spills, blood and flames and, additionally, lets vapors from body sweat pass through. The MB also aids in heat resistance and controls moisture transport. The TL provides comfort and heat resistance and allows metabolic heat release to the environment. The underwear (UV) is worn by Formula One drivers for safety from fuel fires during an accident. The honeycomb (HC) is an insulation material utilized to access its suitability in conjunction with the turnout gear. The physical characteristics of each layer are stated in **Table 2**.

2.2 Experimental results

A permanent skin damage will occur when the temperature of the basal layer exceeds 44°C after a certain exposure duration. Henceforth, to determine the

Outer shell (OS)	Material: Aramid fabric 100% (meta-aramid 80%, para-aramid 20%)	Thickness: 0.40 mm
	Weight: 209 g/m^2	Pattern: Ripstop
Moisture barrier (MB) (substrate + PTFE film)	Material: Meta-aramid 100%(Substrate) + PTFE film	
	Weight: 190 g/m^2	Pattern: Plain weave
	Thickness: 0.347 mm	
Felt insulation of thermal liner (TL)	Material: Meta aramid 100%	
	Weight: 149 g/m^2	
Face cloth of thermal liner (TL)	Material: Meta aramid 100% (Face cloth)	
	Weight: 149 g/m^2	Pattern: Plain weave
	Thickness: 1.754 mm	
Under wear (UW)	Material: Meta aramid 100%	Thickness: 0.61 mm
Honeycomb (HC)	Material: Meta aramid 100%	Thickness: 3 mm

Table 2.
Material properties.

exposure time, experiments are started with an initial guess of 10 seconds. The performance of different layups (Type A, B, and C) was evaluated based on the transmitted flux recorded by the heat flux gauge at the substrate. It was then converted to temperature values using ABAQUS® software. Type A was first exposed to an incident flux of 84 and 126 kW/m^2 for 10 seconds. If the basal layer temperature was estimated to be above 44°C, then types B and C were tested at that exposure time. If not, the exposure time was increased, and the experiment was repeated for type A until the basal layer temperature did not exceed 44°C.

Figure 3(a) displays the skin time-temperature histories for type A, B and C. The basal layer temperature for type A remains below the recommended value of 44°C at 10 and 20 seconds of exposure. However, under an exposure time of 25 seconds, the skin temperature reaches approximately 55°C, which exceeds the threshold value. For type B, the skin temperature remains lower than the threshold value, at around 42°C. In the case of type C, the skin temperature reaches ≈48°C. Based on these results, the three configurations can be ranked as follows: type B performs the best under extreme conditions, followed by type C and then type A.

Figure 3(b) illustrates the skin temperature-time history of type A, B and C for an incident flux of 126 kW/m^2. The type A configuration performed well for an exposure time of up to 15 seconds. However, it failed when the exposure time exceeded 15 seconds. Type B and C configurations, on the other hand, were able to maintain lower skin temperatures, 36% and 31% below the maximum estimated temperature of type A for the basal layer, respectively. In terms of the dermal base, type B performed 18% better and type C performed 14% better than type A. These percentages represent a reduction in skin temperature and an improved level of protection.

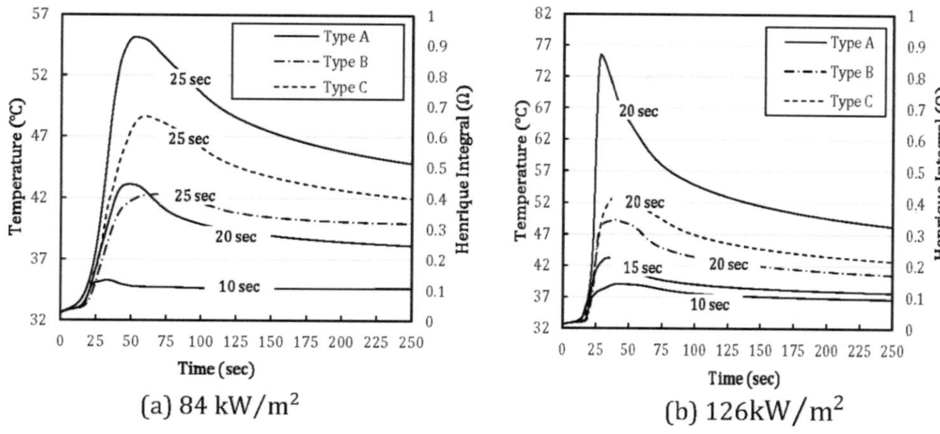

Figure 3.
Skin basal layer temporal-temperature at two levels of heat flux.

2.3 Auxiliar protection significance

The significance of auxiliary layers is estimated based on superficial burn injuries utilizing the Henrique integral [45]. Type B and type C provided more protection by prolonging the time to burn injuries. In the case of type A, no burn was predicted for an incident heat flux of 84 kW/m^2 and 126 kW/m^2 up to an exposure duration of 20 and 15 seconds, respectively. For type A, exposed to 84 kW/m^2 for 25 seconds, a first-degree burn was estimated after 35 seconds and a second-degree burn at 37 seconds. This close gap is associated with rapid increase in skin temperature due to outer shell failure.

Similarly, type A exposed to 126 kW/m^2 for 20 seconds, a second-degree burn was predicted at the 24th second and a third-degree burn at the 74th second. In the case of type B, no burn injuries are projected for 84 kW/m^2; except for an incident flux of 126 kW/m^2 for 20 seconds, a first-degree burn is predicted after 35 seconds. Type C underperformed type B with first-degree burn at the 55th second at 84 kW/m^2 incident flux for an exposure time of 25 seconds and a second-degree burn after 30 seconds for an incident flux of 126 kW/m^2 for 20 seconds of exposure time.

At life-threatening conditions of 126 kW/m^2, it is observed that a second-degree burn will ensue rapidly after a first-degree burn if the outer shell fabric undergoes thermal degradation. Since the Henrique integral is a chemical rate process, it is observed that the underlying tissue in the basal layer does not have enough time to react to extreme temperature variations, so skin tissues undergo chemical changes rapidly, causing second-degree burn immediately. Therefore, an auxiliary protective layer is recommended for firefighters involved in severe fire conditions.

Adding an extra layer to the existing protective suit has proven to mitigate the burn injuries, but care must be taken when the thermal comfort of firefighters is assessed. The use of the honeycomb structure between the moisture barrier and the thermal liner was proven to be beneficial. However, because of the difficulties in retaining its shape during use, it can only be applied to protect the front chest or the back area. It will restrict mobility. As a result, it is not recommended. In comparison, the meta-aramid fabric layer is comfortable and can easily be worn inside an existing suit. Based on this work, the application of type B configuration is recommended.

However, care must be taken while implementing the result of this study to real-life conditions as the assessment was done under laboratory conditions.

Since the study of high thermal-resistant textiles is destructive in nature, numerical techniques are employed to study heat dissipation rates and evaluate other parameters such as moisture effect and superficial burns at variable heat flux levels. These numerical techniques are accurate and cost effective; henceforth, reliable information can be obtained if boundary conditions are rigorously evaluated and applied.

3. Boundary conditions

The protective assembly consists of multiple fabric layers, and the thermal exchange across each layer is affected by a combination of conduction, convection and radiation. Heat energy penetrates the system via thermal radiation. A portion of this is reflected towards the ambient as radiation $\left\{\sigma\varepsilon\left(T_{\text{fab}}^4 - T_{\text{amb}}^4\right)\right\}$ and convection loss $\{h\,(\Delta T)\}$, while most of it is conducted $\left\{k\frac{\partial T}{\partial x}\right\}$ through the fabric. In between fabric layers, the thermal energy is exchanged via net radiation $\left\{\frac{F\sigma}{\frac{1}{\varepsilon_1}-\frac{1}{\varepsilon_2}-1} \times \Delta T^4\right\}$ and conduction/convection. External effects on these boundary conditions should be evaluated to predict heat dissipation rates. In addition, at high flux, smoke layers and boundary and cavity convention are the most important. **Figure 4** illustrates thermal exchange between the fabric layers and with the environment [46].

3.1 Effect of smoke layer

Smoke in the path of radiative rays causes a reduction in the intensity of the radiation. An estimate is made to determine the amount of radiative energy absorbed by the smoke layer. If Nomex® burns completely, it produces heteropolar gases such as CO_2 and H_2O and symmetric diatomic molecular gas N_2 as per the chemical reaction in Eq. (2). N_2 is transparent to electromagnetic waves in the infrared region and does not emit or absorb thermal radiation in its natural state. On the other hand, heteropolar gases absorb and emit radiation in their respective spectral thermal bands.

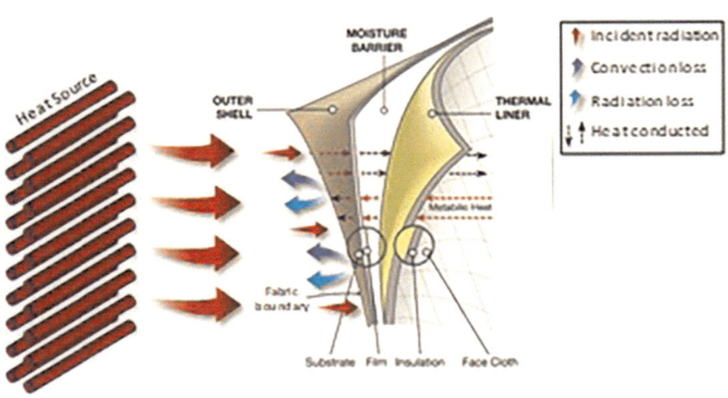

Figure 4.
Thermal exchange in a multi-layered turnout gear.

The "effective emissivity" and "effective absorptivity" of heteropolar gases are evaluated using experimental observation charts developed by Hottel [47, 48]. Precise calculations of absorptivity are complicated, so engineering approximations are used [49].

$$C_{14}H_{10}N_2O_2 + 15.5O_2 + 58.25N_2 \rightarrow 14CO_2 + 5H_2O + 60.27N_2 \quad (2)$$

The volume fraction of CO_2 in combustion products is estimated to be 0.18 and that of H_2O to be 0.06. These volume fractions are based on complete combustion, which is an engineering approximation and would vary at each experimental execution. Therefore, to account for such variations in an ongoing analysis, an optimistic approach was applied, and volume fractions of 0.3 for CO_2 and 0.1 for H_2O were considered [50]. An atmospheric pressure of 1 atm was also assumed for the estimation of partial pressures (P). Absorptivity is estimated based on a relation [48] as below,

$$\alpha_i = \varphi_i \times \varepsilon_i\left(P_i.L, T_g, 1atm\right) \times \frac{T_g^{\varnothing}}{T_s} \quad (3)$$

where, subscript i refers to the participating gas, $L = 2 \times \Delta x$ is the mean beam length, φ_i is the pressure correction factor, T_g is the gas temperature, T_s is the temperature source emitting radiation normal to the radiative surface and $\varnothing$ is a constant value [47], 0.65 for CO_2 and 0.45 H_2O. With the assumption of 1 atmospheric pressure, the correction factor, φ_i, reduces to unity. Overlapping waveband correction $\Delta\varepsilon$ for emissivity estimation of a mixture for a maximum gas thickness of Δx = 0.02 m (assumed from experimental observations) was evaluated. If $\Delta\varepsilon$ is found to be of less significance for this case, it is disregarded in extended calculations. ε_{mix} was estimated as [51],

$$\varepsilon_{mix} = \varphi_{CO_2}.\varepsilon_{CO_2}\left(P_{CO_2}.L, T_g\right) + \varphi_{H_2O}.\varepsilon_{H_2O}\left(P_{H_2O}.L, T_g\right) - \Delta\varepsilon \quad (4)$$

$\Delta\varepsilon$ is evaluated using volume fractions of CO_2 and H_2O as,

$$\begin{gathered}\frac{P_{H_2O}}{P_{CO_2} + P_{H_2O}} = 0.25 \\ P_{CO_2}.L + P_{H_2O}.L \approx 0.016 \ll 1\end{gathered} \quad (5)$$

From Hottel's [47, 48] correction charts $\Delta\varepsilon \approx 0$, thus, Eq. (3) gives,

$$\varepsilon_i(P_i.L) = \int_0^{\Delta x} P_i \times L\, d(\Delta x) \quad (6)$$

The interference of the smoke layer in front of the outer shell under intense exposure to a radiant heat source is dependent on gas layer thickness Δx and source temperature T_s. The gaseous particles attenuate radiative flux passing through, independent of the gas type. The particles of carbon dioxide exhibit stable emissivity, ε_{CO_2}, irrespective of the source temperature, though they have an ascending relationship with increasing smoke layer thickness, Δx. The absorptivity, α_{CO_2}, of carbon dioxide demonstrated a descending relationship to source temperature with constant thickness and ascending relationship with thickness, Δx, of the smoke layer. These relations for carbon dioxide are presented in **Figure 5**. The water vapor's emissivity, ε_{H_2O}, decreases as the source temperature increases with a constant water vapor layer thickness; however, higher emissivity is observed with increased water vapor layer thickness, Δx. A similar trend is observed in the case of water vapor absorptivity, α_{H_2O}, as evident from **Figure 6**.

During pyrolysis, the volume fraction of carbon dioxide is significant compared to water vapor in standard humid conditions, so in theory, its effect on irradiance at the outer shell boundary is more important than water vapor. The expected interference of carbon dioxide particles due to absorption or emission of incident radiative flux is in the range of 0.03–0.055, estimated from **Figure 5**, and that of water vapor is in the range of 0.015–0.035, projected from **Figure 6**. When the heat source was radiating at flux densities of magnitude greater than 41 kW/m^2, the combined effect of heteropolar gases would attenuate the maximum radiative flux by 8.5% and the minimum by 4.5%. An insignificant portion of incident flux density can be safely ignored for the rest of the analysis.

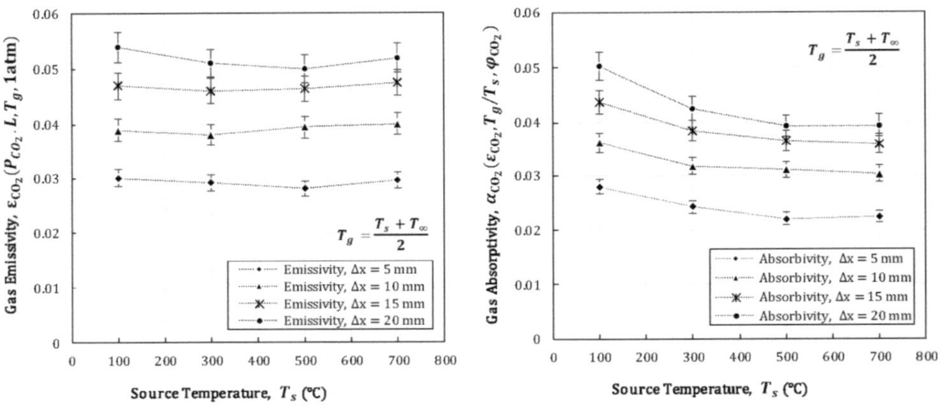

Figure 5.
Carbon-dioxide gas emissivity and absorptivity at variable source temperatures.

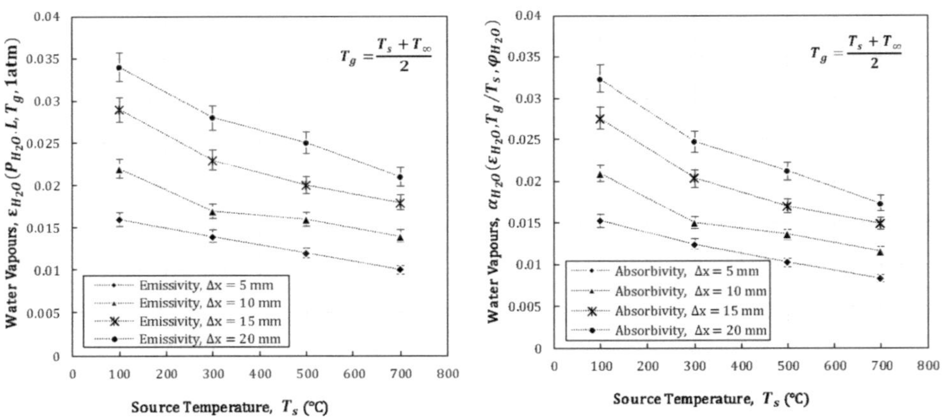

Figure 6.
Water vapor gas emissivity and absorptivity at variable source temperatures.

In conclusion, during pyrolysis, smoke layers up to 20 mm in thickness have little to no interference to irradiance at the outer shell boundary layer for extreme fire conditions.

3.2 Air cavity

The thermal exchange through the air cavity in between fabric layers dictates the dominant mode of heat transfer, that is, convective or conductive. The cavity thickness, δ_s, as per the research prospective is 1–6.35 mm. Based on relation $Ra_{\delta_s} = \frac{g\beta\ (\Delta T)\delta_s}{v^2} \times Pr$, for varying separation distance $\delta_s = 2, 6.35, 10, 20$ and 50 mm, where ΔT is the temperature difference at bounding layers of the air cavity, a dominant mode of heat exchange is estimated. The slave boundary, T_{cold}, is assumed to be at room temperature of 25°C. It is estimated that when cavity thickness is below 6.35 mm, the interface media is purely conductive. **Figure 7** can be utilized to estimate flow behavior at other varying thicknesses.

3.3 Thermal decomposition

The energy released during thermochemical reactions and mass loss rate at the specific temperature ranges were established for each fabric layer, utilizing thermogravimetric analysis (TGA) and High Differential Scanning Calorimetry (HDSC). Linseis model STA PT1000 [52] is utilized. The purpose of TGA and HDSC is to estimate density change and specific heat of the fabric layers at elevated temperatures. During simulation, the algorithm calls in temperature-specific user-defined material properties for each layer, depending on the solution phase (heating or cooling).

From **Figure 8**, for outer shell, the density is estimated to change linearly over time from 522.5 to 458 kg/m^3, valid in a temperature range of 25–125°C, due to evaporation of moisture from the fabric. From 150 to 480°C, it is 442–380 kg/m^3, and from 480 to 720°C, it is 380–27 kg/m^3. For moisture barrier, the temperature ranges as per density change are evaluated as 550.7–522.5 kg/m^3 between 25 and 125°C and 522.5–467 kg/m^3 between 250 and 418°C. In the decomposition temperature range of 418–719°C, it is estimated to be 467–27.5 kg/m^3, linearly. For thermal liner, the density change is estimated to be (−) 15%, as 170–144 kg/m^3 between 25 and 432°C. For Nomex®

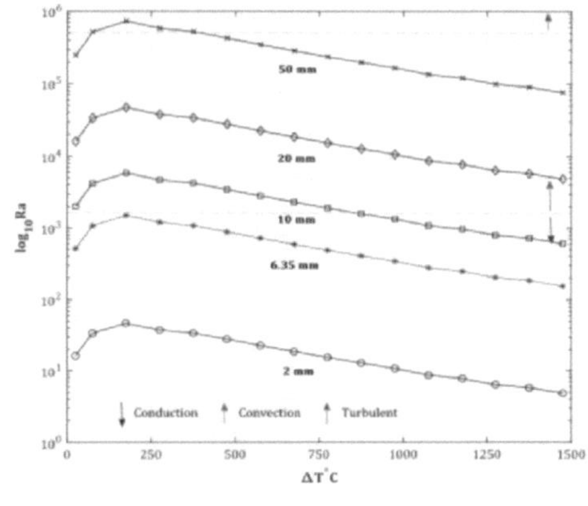

Figure 7.
Flow characteristics at varying cavity thicknesses.

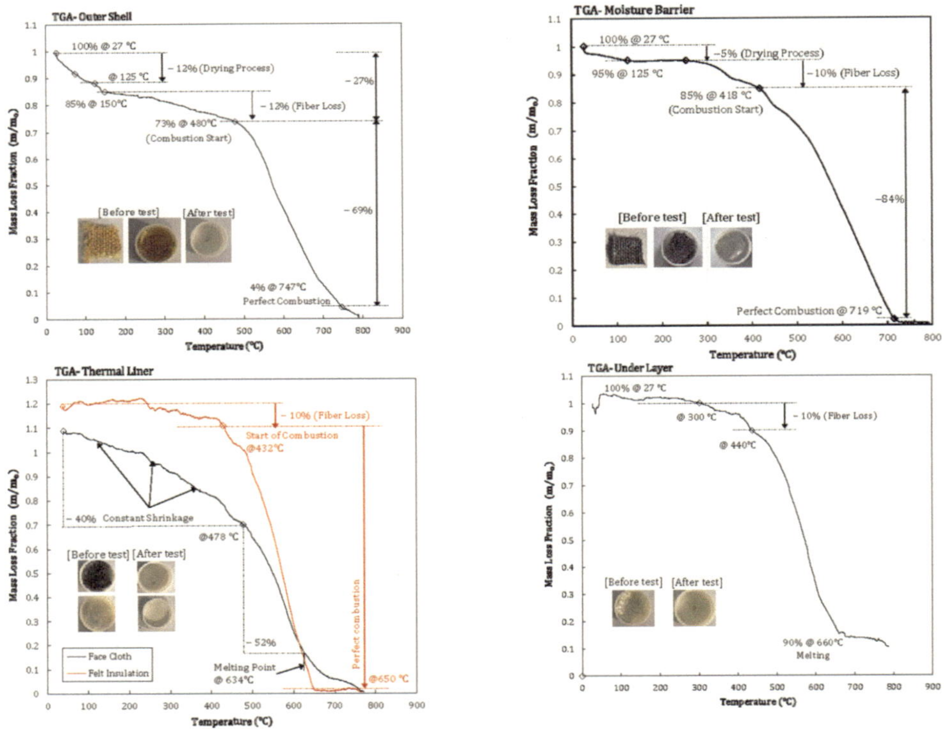

Figure 8.
Thermal gravimetric analysis (TGA) of the turnout gear fabric layers.

under layer, the density is taken as a constant value of 138 kg/m^3 as the temperature is not expected to reach above 300°C.

The concept of apparent specific heat requires the knowledge of temperature ranges and respective specific heat values at those limits. The HDSC analysis for the outer shell is not performed, as the composition is of Nomex®IIIA, and extensive literature is available on the apparent specific heat of it.

In case of the outer shell, the latent energy released due to moisture evaporation between 75 and 125°C and the thermochemical reaction energy released during decomposition between 420 and 700°C is added to the initial value of specific heat during the heating phase. On cooling, the normal specific heat path is followed. Similarly, the density is varied as per mass loss analysis performed on TGA and its implementation to account for decomposition. Henceforth, detailed material properties are shown in **Table 3**. Skin thermal properties have been documented in Ghazy and Bergstrom [53].

4. Numerical model

Numerical models and their validity have been well documented for the prediction of heat dissipation in a single or multi-layered turnout gear for bench-scale studies [42, 49, 50, 54–58]. **Figure 9** represents thermal exchange in between fabric layers in a bench-scale setting. Henceforth, an overview is presented in this section to understand basic mechanics of thermal exchange.

Characteristic	Outer shell	Moisture barrier	Thermal liner	Underlayer
Thickness (m)	0.4×10^{-3}	0.34×10^{-3}	1.75×10^{-3}	0.6×10^{-3}
*Density (kg/m^3)	521–380	170–144	550–27	138–110
*Conductivity (W/m °C)	0.047–0.255	0.047–0.255	0.036	0.047–0.255
*Specific heat (J/kg °C)	1300–2515	1300–2500	1088–2300	1300
Emissivity	0.9	0.9	0.9	0.9

**The thermal properties are dependent on temperature ranges and thermal phase as per TGA and HDSC.*

Table 3.
Fabric material thermal properties.

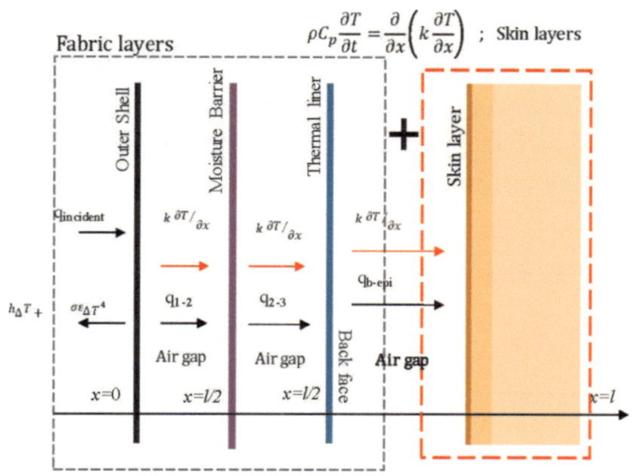

Figure 9.
Thermal exchange between fabric layers in turnout gear.

An energy balance for pure heat exchange between multiple fabric layers can be modeled as per,

$$\rho C_p \frac{\partial T}{\partial t} = \frac{\partial}{\partial x}\left(k \frac{\partial T}{\partial x}\right) + \omega_b \left(\rho C_p\right)\big|_b (T_a - T) + Q_m \tag{7}$$

Conduction across air gap is treated as per Eq. (8), where k_{eff} is the ratio of thermal conductivity of air and its thickness t.

$$k \frac{\partial T}{\partial x} = k_{eff} \frac{\partial T}{\partial x} = \frac{k_{air}}{t_{air}} \frac{\partial T}{\partial x} \tag{8}$$

In between fabric layers, the amount of radiation being transmitted is treated as $q_{rad} = C\left(T_1^4 - T_2^4\right)$ and is dependent on view factor F and emissivity ε, for radiation constant C. Where $C = \frac{F\sigma}{\frac{1}{\varepsilon_1} \frac{1}{\varepsilon_2} 1}$, ω_b is the blood perfusion rate, $kg/m^3 s$, $\left(\rho C_p\right)\big|_b$ is the volumetric heat capacity (blood), $J/m^3.^{\circ}$C, T_a is the arterial temperature/core body, and Q_m is the metabolic heat generation/tissue heat generation rate, W/M^3. Torvi rigorously tested this model and found that the profusion term $\{\omega_b\left(\rho C_p\right)\big|_b(\theta_a - \theta)\}$ had no impact on thermal conductivity of skin in different states [59]. Correlating with Lipkin and Hardy, it takes 20 seconds for the skin to react by increasing blood flow and thus the minimal effect of heat diffusion through it [60]. The emissivity of 0.94 has little effect on skin temperature [61]. Moisture evaporation and carbonization of the skin ensue second- and third-degree burns and can be ignored in the study of burn predictions at high exposures levels.

For thermal manikin, it is necessary to model the incompressible Navier-Stokes equations to simulate large air cavities of more than 10 mm. Limited studies [30, 62, 63] have been done on this as the analysis is time costly with large data points to process. Commercially available software such as ABAQUS® package can be utilized to achieve this task, where air is treated as an incompressible Newtonian fluid. The continuity, momentum and energy equations [64] are all used in this scenario. Detailed study on numerical models have been presented in a recent study [46].

ABAQUS® is employed to model time-dependent thermal behavior. The practical implications influencing numerical solutions are variant. Each layer is distinctive, materially and structurally. The outer shell has a different thickness, texture and material characteristics as opposed to the moisture barrier and thermal liner. The garment interacts with the outside environment and wearer's skin via thermal conduction, convection and radiation. Therefore, moisture significance, burn degree and survival time are studied utilizing numerical approximations based on boundary conditions defined in Section 3.

5. Discussion

5.1 Moisture effect

Moisture can accumulate in firefighter garments during active use, either from an outside source during operation or through perspiration. The latent heat of vaporization, Δh_{er1}, is dependent on the mass fraction of moisture, ϕ, present within the outer shell. The initial moisture mass fraction, ϕ, of 0.05 (5%) [65] is varied to 0.5 (50%), representing partial saturation of the outer shell. The safety offered by convectional protective garment assembly (type A) is then estimated at radiant flux levels of 41, 84 and 126 kW/m^2 for an exposure duration of 25, 25 and 20 seconds as shown in **Figure 10**. The effect of moisture permeation on burn degree with each successive increment of heat flux intensity is presented. The red markers indicate an initial mass fraction of moisture of fabric, that is, 5%, due to a relative humidity of 65%. At a radiant flux of 41 kW/m^2, no burn damage is predicted. However, the temperature of the skin escalates to the threshold level of pain when the moisture content is 5% and 10%, transcribed as "time to pain."

5.2 Superficial burns

Burn degree damage for the basal layer and the dermal base is estimated as shown in **Figure 11**. Subjected to an incident heat flux of 84 kW/m^2 for 25 seconds (Model 1), first-degree burn is observed after 36 seconds, and a second-degree burn is detected after 38 seconds. This minor difference between first and second-degree burns indicates physical failure, also evident with a sharp rise in burn integral Ω. Also, skin temperature T is an exponential function of Ω; as a result, a second-degree burn ensues from a first-degree burn in close approximation. Under exposure of

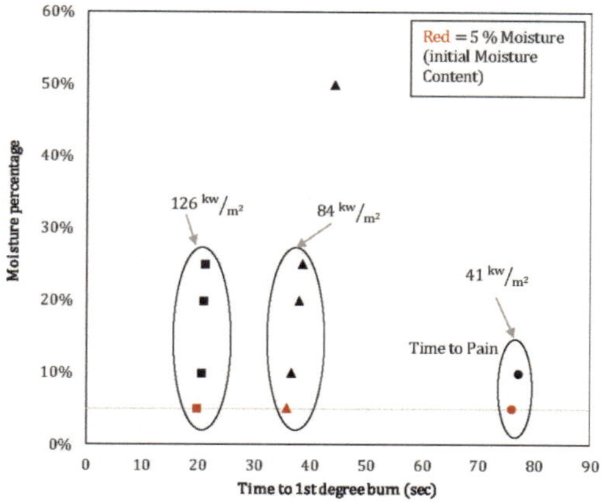

Figure 10.
Moisture effect on first-degree burns.

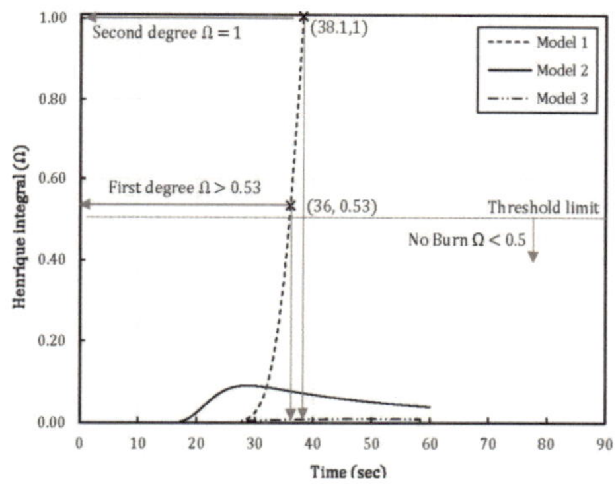

Figure 11.
Approximation of superficial burn degree.

126 kW/m^2 for 15 seconds (Model 2), no superficial degree burn is estimated by Henrique integral evaluation. Under radiant exposures, by the current estimate, a third-degree is highly unlikely, as no third-degree burns for models 1, 2 and 3 are predicted. It is apparent from the present study that garment assembly with an added protective layer protected the wearer from all types of burn injuries and increased thermal efficiency by absorbing additional thermal energy within the auxiliary layer.

5.3 Survival curve

Radiant exposure survival curves are proposed for a heat source ranging from 2.5 to 126 kW/m^2. They represent the modern thermal environment. These curves would be beneficial to estimate the survival time for firefighters wearing an existing multi-layered protective suit. The tolerance time of a firefighter wearing special protective clothing varies depending on the subjected thermal environment. It is argued that those conditions would only occur under circumstances where a firefighter is involuntarily centred due to falling off a burning ceiling or roof [66]. A time-temperature curve was presented in Stoll's work by accessing the damage to naked skin [36]. This curve represented superficial burn damage, and in concurrence with the fabric test, tolerance time from exposure was established by Stoll. Limitations of Stoll's tolerance exposure curve are,

1. Rectangular heat fluxes ranging from 4.2 to 16.8 kW/m^2 were used to establish this criterion, and extrapolation techniques are required for exposure level not considered by Stoll.

2. Assessment of fabric was strictly dependent on the assumption of rectangular heat pulse/source; discrepancy from this shape invalidates the data.

3. A feasibility study on Stoll's curves indicates that it may fail when an extra layer of protection is added, that is, from single fabric to multiple fabrics [67].

The proposed radiant exposure curve addressed these limitations. It utilizes Henrique integral [68] for superficial burn degree evaluation at each successive increment in exposure level. The linear incremental exposure levels selected for this study are "2.5, 10, 20, 41, 60, 84, 100, 115, 126" kW/m^2. An incident radiant heat flux of 2.5 kW/m^2 represents routine working conditions; a value of 10 kW/m^2 represents hazard working conditions; above 10 kW/m^2, they are categorised as emergency working conditions [10, 69, 70]. An incident heat flux of 20 kW/m^2 signifies floor level heat flux for flashover fires [71–74]. The values of 41 and 84 kW/m^2 represent industrial flashfire lower and average heat flux values [7]. They are recommended by international standards for performance evaluation [24, 32, 35]. The value of 126 kW/m^2 is the newly proposed limit for performance evaluation from the current study.

The established radiant exposure curves are plotted in **Figure 12**. The black squared markers represent first-degree burn limit, the red solid line to represent second-degree burn limit, and black circle markers show third-degree burn limit.

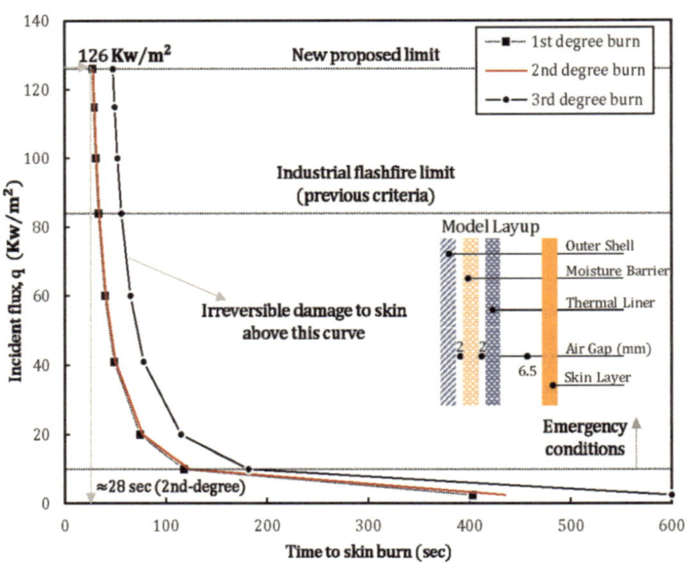

Figure 12.
Radiant exposure survival curve.

It indicates a time to burn damage under several incident heat fluxes for a convectional garment layup.

It is observed from **Figure 12** that the time to skin burn injuries is an exponential function of time, with a linear increase in incident heat flux; the time to burn injuries will proceed at a 100 times faster rate. This behavior is analogous to the rate of injury reported for the naked skin [61]. Effective use of this graph is an extension of Stoll's curve with its limitations addressed. The information extracted from the proposed curves are,

1. A first-degree burn under exposure of current flashfire conditions of 84 kW/m^2 is estimated at 33.6 seconds. For a newly proposed limit of 126 kW/m^2, it is approximated at 27.6 seconds, a 6-second difference.

2. Similarly, a second-degree burn for 84 kW/m^2 and 126 kW/m^2 is estimated at 34.4 and 28.5 seconds, respectively.

3. Irreversible damage to the skin will occur when the exposure duration exceeds 56.2 seconds for 84 kW/m^2 and 47.9 seconds for 126 kW/m^2.

In practical conditions, it is unfeasible for firefighters to gauge their skin temperature without the aid of a thermal sensor. However, the severity of fire can be assessed before engaging it. During operation, the initial indicator of skin burn is the sensation of pain, felt when skin temperature reaches 44°C. The exponential nature of burn damage in skin tissue demonstrates that once the pain is felt, superficial burn injuries will ensue shortly, and in extreme conditions, it will be within seconds. To escape from such a situation without harm, it is important to have knowledge of "survival time." The survival time is defined as a point between the pain threshold and the second-degree curve (blister curve) [36]. In a physical situation, it indicates when pain is felt but blister is not produced. In the current study, this point is determined by considering the first-degree curve as a limitation. Hence, a survival time is estimated by subtracting the time when pain is felt from when a first-degree burn is observed. In **Table 4**, the survival time for a linear increase in incident heat flux for a multi-layered garment is presented.

5.4 Fire-resistant fabrics and sustainability

Textile fabrics, irrespective of their application, will ignite and burn. Fire-resistant fabrics will burn either via flaming combustion (flame contact) or via smoldering (radiant source). Henceforth, protective fabrics are treated with various flame retardants to survive both types of burn. Flame retardants can be categorized into two types: additive and reactive. Additive flame retardants are incorporated into a material or product without forming any bonds or chemical reactions with the product. On the other hand, reactive flame retardants undergo a chemical reaction with the raw materials during the manufacturing process of the final material or product intended for commercial use [75].

In terms of environmental impact, the toxicity of smoke generated due to the burning of additives has implications on its end user, that is, firefighters or military personnel. The different routes of exposure, such as dermal absorption, ingestion (oral) and inhalation, play a role in determining the level of risk posed by a hazardous

Incident flux (kW/m²)	**Time to pain (sec)	*Time to blistering (second-degree burn) (sec)	***Survival time (sec)
2.5	200.0	435.4	203.2
10	89.3	122.8	28.2
20	57.8	76.8	16.4
41	39.2	50.3	9.7
60	32.4	40.9	7.5
84	27.6	34.4	6.0
100	25.4	31.6	5.5
115	23.9	29.7	5.1
126	23.0	28.5	4.9

**Time to second-degree burn from Henrique integral and blistering defined by ASTM C 1055-99. **Time skin temperature reached a value of 44°C defined by ASTM C 1055. ***Survival time defined by Stoll and Chianta [36].*

Table 4.
Survival time estimate under extreme radiant exposure.

substance. US National Research Council Committee on Toxicology summarized 16 key flame retardants or flame-retardant classes for textiles by surveying industries making and/or using flame retardants [76]. They have been detailed in [75], with their relative hazard index concluding that it is less than 1 for all types of exposure routes to public or professional.

Inherently fire-resistant fibers are manufactured by chemically bounding flame retardants to the fiber-forming polymeric molecules or as an additive in the structure. Henceforth, the potential toxicity is limited during manufacturing and during disposal at the end-of-life cycle. Below are such fibers with their sustainability towards the environment [77],

Polyester: The manufacturer of these products claims that they possess environmentally friendly characteristics. During their manufacturing process, no emissions or waste products are generated, and they are cost-effective to clean. Trevira fiber and filament yarns have the potential to meet the criteria for the Oeko-Tex 100 Certificate/eco-label, which signifies that they do not contain any harmful substances.

Modacrylics: They have been in existence for over half a century and are categorized as polymers capable of forming fibers. These polymers are derived from resins that consist of copolymers of acrylonitrile. Acrylonitrile units make up a minimum of 35% but less than 85% of the resin's weight ($\pm CH_2CH[CN]\pm$), while another comonomer like vinyl chloride, vinylidene chloride or vinyl bromide is also present. Vinylidene chloride is a comonomer, and to enhance flame resistance, antimony trioxide may be incorporated into the resin before it undergoes wet or dry spinning. Alternatively, vinyl bromide can be utilized as a comonomer. At present, there are only a limited number of commercially available modacrylic fibers, with Kanecaron (manufactured by Kaneka Corporation) being a notable example, which is based on vinylidene chloride/antimony oxide. However, concerns have been raised regarding the presence of both halogen and antimony in these fibers, casting doubt on their future economic viability.

Polypropylene: Prior to the melt spinning of polypropylene fiber, additives, including both halogen and non-halogen types, are introduced into the molten mixture. Examples of these additives include Sandoflam 5072 (manufactured by Clariant) and Ciba® Flamestab® NOR™ 116.

Aromatic polyamide: Two prominent commercial examples of para-aramids and meta-aramids are manufactured by DuPont as Kevlar® and Nomex®. The primary environmental concerns associated with these materials arise from the challenges involved in disposing of both manufacturing waste and end-of-life waste. However, their high value encourages recycling efforts. During the manufacturing process, the potential toxicity of intermediates has also posed a significant challenge. Specifically, Kevlar® is synthesized using the monomers 1,4-phenylene-diamine (also known as para-phenylenediamine) and terephthaloyl chloride through a condensation reaction that produces hydrochloric acid as a by-product. This reaction results in liquid-crystalline behavior and a mechanical drawing, causing the polymer chains to align along the fiber's direction. Initially, hexamethylphosphoramide (HMPA) was used as the solvent for polymerization. However, toxicology testing revealed that HMPA caused tumors in the noses of rats. As a result, DuPont discontinued the use of HMPA and switched to a different solvent, which is a mixture of *N*-methyl-pyrrolidone and calcium chloride.

Polymelamine fiber: Basofil® (manufactured by BASF) is a heat and flame-resistant fiber that utilizes patented melamine technology. According to the manufacturer, Basofil® fiber complies with all environmental regulations pertaining to its processing and use. It possesses a Limiting Oxygen Index (LOI) value of 32, has low thermal conductivity, exhibits excellent heat dimensional stability and does not shrink, melt, or drip when exposed to flames. Although Basofil® fiber is relatively weak, it can be processed using standard textile machinery to create woven, knit and nonwoven fabrics. It is also suitable for producing batting or fabric fire barriers for mattresses and upholstered furniture. Like aramids, the disposal of Basofil® fiber after use presents an environmental challenge.

Non-toxic phosphorus fire resistant (FR) solutions such as EDA-DOPO (ED) and DOPO-PEPA (DP) were applied to polyethylene terephthalate (PET), replacing halogenated FR solutions [78]. The DOPO-based FR solution passed the vertical burning test, making it a suitable candidate for future application. Other studies have focused on developing carbon fiber-reinforced composites engineered with renewable compounds [79]. These bio-based organic compounds are combined with a renewable monomer, the triglycidyl ether of phloroglucinol (TGPh), with hexahydro-4-methylphthalic anhydride (HMPA), resulting in exceptional intrinsic flame resistance. Bio-composite applications to produce eco-friendly FR with renewable materials have proven to have a significant impact in lowering environmental footprint. Such impact has been discussed in a review study published by Madyaratri et al. [80]. Several recent studies have also proven this concept such as for cotton fabric [81, 82], aerogels linked with biobased cationic amylopectin derivative for extreme temperature conditions [83, 84] and glass fiber composite [85].

The utilization of flame retardants offers advantages to both society and the environment. While it is true that not all flame retardants, past or future, can be deemed completely safe from all perspectives, the application of proper scientific knowledge and regulatory measures can effectively prevent the distribution of hazardous substances to consumers. Nonetheless, it is crucial to recognize that flame retardants, as a group, significantly enhance fire safety by reducing the likelihood of ignition, minimizing heat release and decreasing the levels of smoke, combustion by-products and harmful environmental toxins.

6. Conclusion

The chapter highlights the significance of fire impact on the individual such as firefighters or military personnel. Emerging new evidence suggests that there is a need to redefine the upper limit of heat flux, which is 84 kW/m^2, which has been the same for the last four decades. Evident from modern construction trends and experimental studies on compartment fires in the past two decades reported an increasing heat flux trend with an average of 150 kW/m^2. Presently, the convectional turnout gear does not offer adequate thermal protection at 126 kW/m^2; henceforth, auxiliary protection measures and a realistic increase of 126 kW/m^2 in the upper limit for testing is recommended. Fire-resistant fabric implications on sustainability in terms of toxicity and end-of-life cycle are a challenging research area. A balance is needed to meet the demand for functionality along with the protection offered by flame retardants. Nevertheless, biobased composites and renewable monomers are being researched to replace conventional halogenated and toxic flame retardants.

Author details

Rumeel Ahmad Bhutta and Sengkwan Choi*
Ulster University, Belfast, United Kingdom

*Address all correspondence to: s.choi@ulster.ac.uk

References

[1] Bajaj P, Sengupta AK. Protective clothing. Textile Progress. 1992;**22**(2–4): 1-110. DOI: 10.1080/004051692086 88856

[2] Mandal S, Annaheim S, Pitts T, Camenzind M, Rossi RM. Studies of the thermal protective performance of fabrics under fire exposure: From small-scale to hexagon tests. Textile Research Journal. 2018;**88**(20):2339-2352. DOI: 10.1177/0040517517723020

[3] Bajaj P. Fire-retardant materials. Bulletin of Materials Science. 1992;**15**(1): 67-76. DOI: 10.1007/BF02745218

[4] Bourbigot S, Flambard X. Heat resistance and flammability of high performance fibres: A review. Fire and Materials. 2002;**26**(4–5):155-168. DOI: 10.1002/fam.799

[5] Yoda N. Studies of the structure and properties of aromatic polyamide. I. Physical properties of poly(m-xylyleneadipamide). Bulletin of the Chemical Society of Japan. 1962; **35**(8):1349-1353. DOI: 10.1246/ bcsj.35.1349

[6] Tsvetkov VN, Shtennikova IN. Structure and rigidity of molecules of aromatic polyamides in solutions. Macromolecules. 1978;**11**(2): 306-312

[7] Behnke WP. Predicting flash fire protection of clothing from laboratory tests using second-degree burn to rate performance. Fire and Materials. 1984; **8**(2):57-63. DOI: 10.1002/fam.8100 80202

[8] Song G, Mandal S, Rossi RM. Thermal Protective Clothing for Firefighters. Duxford, United Kingdom: Woodhead Publishing; 2017

[9] Rossi R. Fire fighting and its influence on the body. Ergonomics. 2003;**46**(10): 1017-1033. DOI: 10.1080/ 0014013031000121968

[10] Abbott NJ, Schulman S. Protection from fire: Nonflammable fabrics and coatings. Journal of Coated Fabrics. 1976; **6**(1):48-64. DOI: 10.1177/152808377600 600106

[11] Elkins W, Thompson JG. Instrumented Thermal Mannikin. NTIS Report No. AD-781 176; 1973

[12] Krasny J, Rockett JA, Huang D. Protecting fire fighters exposed in room fires: Comparison of results of bench scale test for thermal protection and conditions during room flashover. Fire Technology. 1988;**24**(1):5-19. DOI: 10.1007/BF01039637

[13] Torvi DA, Hadjisophocleus GV. Research in protective clothing for firefighters: State of the art and future directions. Fire Technology. 1999;**35**(2): 111-130. DOI: 10.1023/A:1015411804979

[14] Hakkarainen T, Oksanen T. Fire safety assessment of wooden facades. Fire and Materials. 2002;**26**(1):7-27. DOI: 10.1002/fam.780

[15] Hakkarainen T. Post-flashover fires in light and heavy timber construction compartments. Journal of Fire Sciences. 2002;**20**(2):133-175. DOI: 10.1177/ 0734904102020002074

[16] Manzello SL, Gann RG, Kukuck SR, Prasad K, Jones WW. Real fire performance of partition assemblies. Fire and Materials. 2005;**29**(6):351-366. DOI: 10.1002/fam.892

[17] Welch S, Jowsey A, Deeny S, Morgan R, Torero JL. BRE large

compartment fire tests-characterising post-flashover fires for model validation. Fire Safety Journal. 2007;**42**(8):548-567. DOI: 10.1016/j.firesaf.2007.04.002

[18] Hwang CH, Lock A, Bundy M, Johnsson E, Ko GH. Effects of fuel location and distribution on full-scale underventilated compartment fires. Journal of Fire Sciences. 2011;**29**(1): 21-52. DOI: 10.1177/07349 04110372119

[19] Bwalya A, Gibbs E, Lougheed G, Kashef A. Heat release rates of modern residential furnishings during combustion in a room calorimeter. Fire and Materials. 2015;**39**(8):685-716. DOI: 10.1002/fam.2259

[20] Marske RA. Characteristics of New Housing - Data.gov. Maryland, USA: US Census Bureau, Department of Commerce; 2016

[21] Kerber S. Analysis of changing residential fire dynamics and its implications on firefighter operational timeframes. Fire Technology. 2012; **48**(4):865-891. DOI: 10.1007/ s10694-011-0249-2

[22] Fenichell S. Plastic: The Making of a Synthetic Century. Michigan, USA: Harper Business; 1996. p. 356

[23] BS EN ISO 13506-1:2017. Protective Clothing Against Heat and Flame. Test Method for Complete Garments. Measurement of Transferred Energy Using an Instrumented Manikin. London, United Kingdom: BSI Standards Publication; 2017

[24] BS EN ISO 17492:2003. Clothing for Protection Against Heat and Flame. Determination of Heat Transmission on Exposure to Both Flame and Radiant Heat. London, United Kingdom: BSI Standard Publications; 2003

[25] Behnke WP. Thermal protective performance test for clothing. Fire Technology. 1977;**13**(1):6-12. DOI: 10.1007/BF02338881

[26] PyroMan™ | Textile Protection and Comfort Center | NC State University. 2019

[27] Norton MJT, Kadolph SJ, Johnson RF, Jordan KA. Design, construction, and use of Minnesota woman, a thermally instrumented mannequin. Textile Research Journal. 1985;**55**(1):5-12. DOI: 10.1177/ 004051758505500102

[28] Trent LC, Resch WA, Coppari LA, Finley DL. Design and construction of a thermally-instrumented mannequin for measuring the burn injury potential of wearing apparel. Textile Research Journal. 1979;**49**(11):639-647. DOI: 10.1177/004051757904901104

[29] Song G. Clothing air gap layers and thermal protective performance in single layer garment. Journal of Industrial Textiles. 2007;**36**(3):193-205. DOI: 10.1177/1528083707069506

[30] Wang Y, Wang Z, Zhang X, Wang M, Li J. CFD simulation of naked flame manikin tests of fire proof garments. Fire Safety Journal. 2015;**71**: 187-193. DOI: 10.1016/j.firesaf.2014. 11.020

[31] BS EN ISO 9151. Protective Clothing Against Heat and Flame—Determination of Heat Transmission on Exposure to Flame. London, United Kingdom: BSI Standards Publication; 2016

[32] BS EN ISO:6942. Protective Clothing—Protection against Heat and Fire—Method of Test: Evaluation of Materials and Material Assemblies When Exposed to a Source of Radiant Heat.

London, United Kingdom: BSI Standard Publications; 2015

[33] ASTM F2702-15. Standard Test Method for Radiant Heat Performance of Flame Resistant Clothing Materials with Burn Injury Prediction. Pennsylvania, USA: American Society for Testing and Materials; 2015

[34] ASTM F2703-08. Standard Test Method for Unsteady-State Heat Transfer Evaluation of Flame Resistant Materials for Clothing with Burn Injury Prediction. Pennsylvania, USA: American Society for Testing of Materials; 2013

[35] NFPA:1971. Standard on Protective Ensembles for Structural Fire Fighting and Proximity Fire Fighting. Quincy, MA: National Fire Protection Association; 2018

[36] Stoll AM, Chianta MA. A Method and Rating System for Evaluation of Thermal Protection. Pennsylvania, USA: Naval Air Development Center Warminster PA Aerospace Medical Research Department; 1968

[37] Henriques FC. Studies of thermal injury; the predictability and the significance of thermally induced rate processes leading to irreversible epidermal injury. Archives of Pathology. 1947;**43**(5):489-502

[38] Weaver JA, Stoll AM. Mathematical Model of Skin Exposed to Thermal Radiation. Warminster: Naval Air Development Center; 1967

[39] Kang S, Kwon M, Choi JY, Choi S. Development of testing environment for thermal protective clothing at critical conditions. In: The Proceedings of 11th Asia-Oceania Symposium on Fire Science and Technology. Singapore: Springer Singapore; 2020. pp. 435-449. DOI: 10.1007/978-981-32-9139-3_32

[40] Psikuta A, Frackiewicz-Kaczmarek J, Frydrych I, Rossi R. Quantitative evaluation of air gap thickness and contact area between body and garment. Textile Research Journal. 2012;**82**(14): 1405-1413. DOI: 10.1177/ 0040517512436823

[41] Li X, Wang Y, Lu Y. Effects of body postures on clothing air gap in protective clothing. Journal of Fiber Bioengineering and Informatics. 2011;**4**(3):277-283. DOI: 10.3993/jfbi09201107

[42] Mell WE, Lawson JR. A heat transfer model for firefighters' protective clothing. Fire Technology. 2000;**36**(1): 39-68. DOI: 10.1023/A:1015429820426

[43] Bhutta RA, Choi S. Thermo-physical evaluation of firefighter outer garment in high flux environments. Textile Research Journal. 2022;**92**(13–14): 2461-2475. DOI: 10.1177/ 00405175221086043

[44] Song G. Modeling Thermal Protection Outfits for Fire Exposures [PhD thesis]. North Carolina, USA: North Carolina State University; 2003

[45] Bhutta RA, Choi S. Mitigation of firefighters' skin burn injuries utilizing auxiliary measures. Textile Research Journal. 2023;**93**(11-12):2775-2788. DOI: 10.1177/00405175221147245/ ASSET/IMAGES/LARGE/10.1177_ 00405175221147245-FIG12.JPEG

[46] Bhutta RA, Choi S. Thermal Protective Performance of Turnout Gear at High Heat Flux Intensity [Thesis]. Belfast, Northern Ireland: Ulster University; 2022

[47] Hottel HC. Heat transmission by radiation from non-luminous gases[1]. Industrial and Engineering Chemistry. 1927;**19**(8):888-894

[48] Modest MF. Radiative Heat Transfer. Oxford, United Kingdom: Elsevier Science; 2013. 882 p

[49] Torvi DA, Dale JD. Heat transfer in thin fibrous materials under high heat flux. Fire Technology. 1999;**35**(3): 210-231. DOI: 10.1023/A:1015 484426361

[50] Torvi DA. Heat Transfer in Thin Fibrous Materials under High Heat Flux Conditions [Ph.D. thesis]. Edmonton, Alberta: University of Alberta; 1997

[51] Kreith F, Manglik R, Bohn M. Principles of Heat Transfer. 7th ed. Stamford, USA: Cengage Learning; 2012

[52] Linseis STA PT 1000: Combined TGA and DSC Measurements. 2020

[53] Ghazy A, Bergstrom DJ. Numerical simulation of transient heat transfer in a protective clothing system during a flash fire exposure. Numerical Heat Transfer; Part A: Applications. 2010;**58**(9): 702-724. DOI: 10.1080/10407782.2010. 516691

[54] Ismail M, Ammar AS, El-Okeily M. Heat transfer through textile fabrics: Mathematical model. Applied Mathematical Modelling. 1988;**12**(4): 434-440. DOI: 10.1016/0307-904X(88) 90075-3

[55] Farnworth B. Mechanisms of heat flow through clothing insulation. Textile Research Journal. 1983;**53**(12): 717-725. DOI: 10.1177/0040517583 05301201

[56] Chen YN. Transient Heat and Moisture Transfer through Thermally Irradiated Clothing. Cambridge, Massachusetts, USA: Massachusetts Institute of Technology; 1959

[57] Torvi DA, Dale JD. Effects of variations in thermal properties on the performance of flame resistant fabrics for flash fires. Textile Research Journal. 1998;**68**(11):787-796. DOI: 10.1177/ 004051759806801102

[58] Lawson JR, Twilley WH. Development of an Apparatus for Measuring the Thermal Performance of Fire Fighters' Protective Clothing. Gaithersburg, USA: U.S. Department of Commerce, Technology Administration, National Institute of Standards and Technology; 1999

[59] Torvi DA, Dale JD. A finite element model of skin subjected to a flash fire. Journal of Biomechanical Engineering. 1994;**116**(3):250. DOI: 10.1115/1. 2895727

[60] Lipkin M, Hardy JD. Measurement of some thermal properties of human tissues. Journal of Applied Physiology. 1954;**7**(2):212-217. DOI: 10.1152/ jappl.1954.7.2.212

[61] Stoll AM, Greene LC. Relationship between pain and tissue damage due to thermal radiation. Journal of Applied Physiology. 1959;**14**(3):373-382. DOI: 10.1152/jappl.1959.14.3.373

[62] Jiang YY, Yanai E, Nishimura K, Zhang H, Abe N, Shinohara M, et al. An integrated numerical simulator for thermal performance assessments of firefighters' protective clothing. Fire Safety Journal. 2010;**45**(5):314-326. DOI: 10.1016/j.firesaf.2010.06.003

[63] Tian M, Wang Z, Li J. 3D numerical simulation of heat transfer through simplified protective clothing during fire exposure by CFD. International Journal of Heat and Mass Transfer. 2016;**93**: 314-321. DOI: 10.1016/j. ijheatmasstransfer.2015.09.027

[64] ABAQUS/Standard User's Manual, Version 6.10. RI: Dassault Systems Simulia Corporation, Providence, USA. 2010

[65] Nomex Fibre Technical Guide. Wilmington, USA: DuPont de Nemours, Incorporation; 2020

[66] Barker R. A Review of Gaps and Limitations in Test Methods for First Responder Protective Clothing and Equipment. National Institute for Occupational Safety and Health (NIOSH); 2005

[67] Zhai LN, Li J. Prediction methods of skin burn for performance evaluation of thermal protective clothing. Burns. 2015; **41**(7):1385-1396. DOI: 10.1016/j.burns.2015.02.019

[68] Henriques FC Jr, Moritz AR. Studies of thermal injury: I. The conduction of heat to and through skin and the temperatures attained therein. A theoretical and an experimental investigation. The American Journal of Pathology. 1947;**23**(4):530

[69] Coletta GC, Arons IJ, Ashley LE, Drennan AP. The Development of Criteria for Firefighters' Gloves Volume II: Glove Criteria and Test Methods. Cambridge, Massachusetts: Arthur D. Little, Inc.; 1976

[70] Foster JA. Measurements of the firefighting environment. Fire Engineers Journal. 1995;**44**(178):30-34

[71] Quintiere JG, Mccaffrey BJ. The Burning of Wood and Plastic Cribs in an Enclosure: Volume 1. Washington, DC, USA: National Bureau of Standards, NBSIR 80-2054; 1980

[72] Thomas PH. Testing products and materials for their contribution to flashover in rooms. Fire and Materials. 1981;**5**(3):103-111. DOI: 10.1002/fam.810050305

[73] Fang JB, Breese JN. Fire Development in Residential Basement Rooms. Washington, DC, USA: National Bureau of Standards. NBSIR 80-2120; 1980. DOI: 10.6028/NBS.IR.80-2120

[74] Babrauskas V. Combustion of Mattresses Exposed to Flaming Ignition Sources: Part 1. Full-Scale Tests and Hazard Analysis. Washington, DC, USA: National Bureau of Standards, NBSIR 77-1290; 1977. DOI: 10.6028/NBS.IR.77-1290

[75] Kinlinc FS. Safety, health and environmental aspects of flame retardants. In: Handbook of Fire Resistant Textiles. Cambridge, UK: Woodhead Publishing; 2013. pp. 108-173

[76] Gardiner DE (chair), Borzelleca DW, Gaylor S, Green R, Horrocks MA, Jayjock S et al. Toxicological Risks of Selected Flame-Retardant Chemicals. 2000

[77] Lowell Center for Sustainable Products. Decabromodiphenylether: An Investigation of Non-Halogenated Substitutes in Electronic Enclosures and Textile Applications. 2005

[78] Özer MS, Wesemann MJ, Gaan S. Flame retardant back-coated PET fabric with DOPO-based environmentally friendly formulations. Progress in Organic Coatings. 2023;**175**:107363. DOI: 10.1016/j.porgcoat.2022.107363

[79] Dinu R, Lafont U, Damiano O, Orange F, Mija A. Recyclable, repairable, and fire-resistant high-performance carbon fiber biobased epoxy. ACS Applied Polymer Materials. 2022;**5**(4): 2542-2552. DOI: 10.1021/

ACSAPM.2C02184/SUPPL_FILE/AP2C02184_SI_001.PDF

[80] Madyaratri EW, Ridho MR, Aristri MA, Lubis MAR, Iswanto AH, Nawawi DS, et al. Recent advances in the development of fire-resistant biocomposites—A review. Polymers. 2022;**14**:362. DOI: 10.3390/polym14030362

[81] Rao W, Shi J, Yu C, Zhao HB, Wang YZ. Highly efficient, transparent, and environment-friendly flame-retardant coating for cotton fabric. Chemical Engineering Journal. 2021;**424**:130556. DOI: 10.1016/j.cej.2021.130556

[82] Li P, Liu C, Xu YJ, Jiang ZM, Liu Y, Zhu P. Novel and eco-friendly flame-retardant cotton fabrics with lignosulfonate and chitosan through LbL: Flame retardancy, smoke suppression and flame-retardant mechanism. Polymer Degradation and Stability. 2020;**181**:109302. DOI: 10.1016/j.polymdegradstab.2020.109302

[83] Ye DD, Wang T, Liao W, Wang H, Zhao HB, Wang YT, et al. Ultrahigh-temperature insulating and fire-resistant aerogels from cationic amylopectin and clay via a facile route. ACS Sustainable Chemistry and Engineering. 2019;**7**(13):11582-11592. DOI: 10.1021/acssuschemeng.9b01487

[84] Xia Z, Kiratitanavit W, Facendola P, Thota S, Yu S, Kumar J, et al. Fire resistant polyphenols based on chemical modification of bio-derived tannic acid. Polymer Degradation and Stability. 2018;**153**:227-243. DOI: 10.1016/J.POLYMDEGRADSTAB.2018.04.020

[85] Laskoski M, Shepherd AR, Mahzabeen W, Clarke JS, Keller TM, Sorathia U. Sustainable, fire-resistant phthalonitrile-based glass fiber composites. Journal of Polymer Science, Part A: Polymer Chemistry. 2018;**56**(11):1128-1132. DOI: 10.1002/pola.28989

Chapter 8

Human Body Temperature Circadian Rhythm in Health and Disease

Ivayla I. Geneva

Abstract

Human body temperature continues to be of interest to researchers with the newest discovery that it had been steadily decreasing since the mid-1800s, thus affecting our definition of normothermia and the cutoff for fever. Further, body temperature constitutes an explicit manifestation of our circadian rhythm, with temperature trough occurring in early morning and peak in the evening in healthy individuals. On the other hand, human illness, as seen among patients ranging from stable hospitalized ones to the critically ill, was shown to correlate with disturbance or even complete disappearance of the body temperature circadian rhythm. Also, night shift work affects the rhythm and had been associated with increased risk for malignancies, gastroenterological and metabolic disorders. Importantly, quantification of the observed rhythm deviations appears to have diagnostic and prognostic value in medicine. This chapter reviews the determinants of body temperature and the body temperature circadian rhythm, discusses the most prominent published research on associations between the rhythm and human disease, and concludes by outlining possible new research avenues and promising clinical applications in the field of chronotherapy.

Keywords: circadian rhythm, body temperature, chronotherapy, fever, hypothermia, personalized medicine

1. Introduction

The circadian rhythm of humans and other living beings had intrigued scientists and philosophers since antiquity. While its first known manifestation was the sleep-wake cycle, over the centuries additional body functions were identified as being controlled by the circadian rhythm. This chapter explores the relationship between human body temperature and our circadian rhythm, which turns out to be one of interdependence. The existing literature is reviewed with a particular emphasis on the health-related effects triggered by disruptions in the diurnal body temperature oscillations. The chapter concludes by offering possible future research avenues that could lead to the development of clinical tools such as mortality prediction models, sepsis early-warning systems and chronotherapy approaches to night shift work-associated disorders and psychiatric illnesses, all based on monitoring body temperature variations.

2. Human body temperature: An evolving story

Human body temperature had been of interest to ancient healers [1–4]. In more recent times, the German physician and researcher Carl Reinhold August Wunderlich became known as the father of clinical thermometry for his pioneering application of a thermometer to measure a precise body temperature. In his 1868 seminal paper [5], Wunderlich used over a million axillary temperature readings from over 25,000 patients to established the first normothermia average point of 37°C, with the upper limit of normal being 38°C. To date, we still use these numbers as a reference standard. Since human body temperature continues to be regarded as an important screening and prognostic tool in modern medicine, further efforts had taken place to establish normothermia ranges and determine the factors that influence body temperature measurements, as was recently review by our group [6].

An important difference in normothermia exists between what are regarded as core body temperature measurement sites (e.g., rectal and transurethral) and the non-core sites such as oral, axillary, or tympanic. The former yield higher temperature measurements than the latter, likely due to heat-dissipating processes like convection occurring at the body surface. **Figure 1** (adopted with modifications and permission from Geneva et al. [6]) illustrates this difference using data from 36 unique peer-reviewed studies. Further, age is a known major determinant of human body temperature, where a decline in temperature is observed as we get older, which is featured in **Figure 2** (adopted with modifications and permission from Geneva et al. [6]). Some studies have shown that body temperature also depends on the subject's sex due to the change in body temperature among pre-menopausal women based on when the measurement is taken with regards to their menstrual cycle [5, 7–9]. In addition, the seasonal environmental temperature itself appears to influence our body temperature – a large study of over 93,000 emergency department patients demonstrated that on average human body temperature is lower by 0.2°C (using temporal artery thermometers) in the winter compared with the summer [10]—a statistically significant difference albeit a small one. Certainly, medical illnesses such as infections, malignancies, thyroid disorders, among many others, can strongly affect our temperature as well.

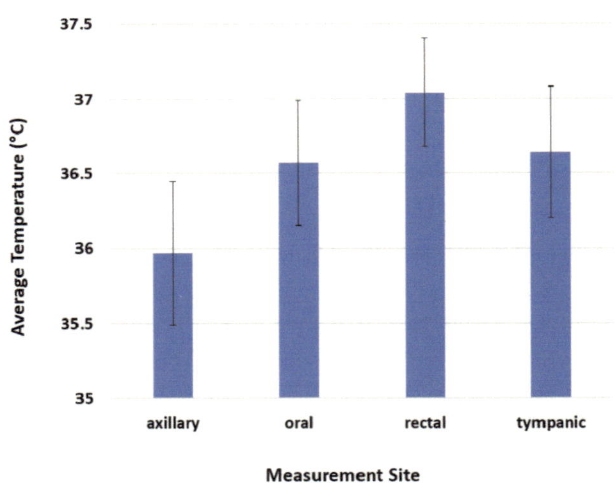

Figure 1.
Human body temperature of healthy volunteers classified by measurement site. Adapted with modifications and with permission from Geneva et al. [6] ***Figure 1B.***

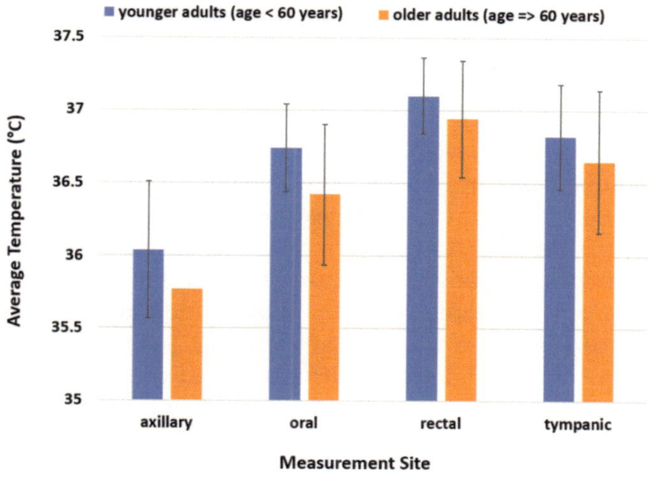

Figure 2.
Human body temperature of healthy volunteers classified by age and measurement site. Adapted with modifications and with permission from Geneva et al. [6] ***Figure 1C.***

Interestingly, the 37°C normothermia average standard had been challenged by several research groups including Obermeyer et al. [11], Diamond et al. [12] and Corsi et al. [13], where a lower non-core average body temperature of 36.6°C, 36.1°C and 36.71°C were reported, respectively. While these findings were based on diverse cohorts and constituted only a point-in-time observation, Protsiv et al. [14] carried out a longitudinal study, where the measurements were adjusted for age, weight, height, and for some data sets for time of the day as well. By combining data from Civil War Union Army veterans covering 1860–1940, the National Health and Nutrition Examination Survey I covering 1971–1975, and the Stanford Translational Research Integrated Database Environment covering 2007–2017, Protsiv et al. discovered a curious trend of steady body temperature decrease at a rate of 0.03°C per birth cohort, leading to a difference of 0.56°C between males born in the 19th century and adult males today; for females, the total decrease was smaller — 0.32°C. Speculative explanations for this discovery centered around two major factors. First, there had been a decrease in metabolism as each new generation is believed to be significantly more sedentary than the prior and most homes are heated in winter and cooled in the summer, thus decreasing the human body basic metabolic rate expenditures. Second, the prevalence of fever in the human population induced by chronic inflammation had declined with the advent and widespread use of antibiotics, vaccines, and non-steroidal anti-inflammatory drugs.

In conclusion and knowing that we currently live in the era of personalized medicine, it is necessary to point out that ultimately, no matter what the population-wide average body temperature is, each person has their own baseline body temperature, which may be several standard deviations above or below the population average. This is illustrated by measured intrapersonal standard deviation of 0.32°C [12] and 0.39°C to 0.4°C [15] in healthy adults, while the range of measured interpersonal body temperatures in the same research studies spanned 2–3°C. This realization prompted several researchers to propose that "one size does not fit all" as it comes to normal body temperature [12, 13]. The definition of normothermia is further complicated by the fact that even within the same organism body temperature changes in a cyclic manner with a period of approximately 24 hours – the circadian rhythm of body temperature, which is the focus of the next chapter section.

3. Diurnal variation of human body temperature – A manifestation of our circadian rhythm

From unicellular organisms to complex mammals like humans, a circadian rhythm exists, whose role revolves around optimizing the function of the organism relative to an approximately 24-hour-long diurnal period [16–20]. While there are many bodily functions that appear to be governed by the circadian rhythm such as sleep, cardiovascular function, respiration, coagulation, and others, as detailed in other chapters of this book, body temperature is one of if not the most easily accessible manifestation of the circadian rhythm. Body temperature can be measured with both good accuracy [21] and at high frequency [22], thus allowing for relatively inexpensive experimental designs in the fields of circadian rhythm and chronotherapy research.

The relationship between body temperature diurnal oscillations and the circadian rhythm was first reported in the 1800s by Davy [23] and Ogle [24]. Currently, we know that in healthy humans the minimum body temperature (the bathyphase) occurs in the early morning about 2 hours before wakening (i.e., 5–7 AM) and the maximum body temperature (the acrophase) occurs in the evening about 2 hours before falling asleep (i.e., 8–10 PM) [25–28]. The body temperature diurnal cycle can be approximated by a sinusoidal curve, whose amplitude is one-half of the total diurnal temperature change (acrophase minus bathyphase), and whose mesor is the rhythm-adjusted mean. The reader can refer to **Figure 3** for an illustration of this cycle. In humans, the amplitude had been measured to be around 0.2–0.8°C [16, 26, 27, 29]. There appear to be certain sex-based differences in the diurnal body temperature cycle just like there were differences in average body temperature between the sexes, as was described in the previous section of this chapter. For instance, Cain et al. [27] showed that on average the bathyphase in healthy women occurred earlier (at 4:46 AM) compared with healthy males (at 6:11 AM). The same study also measured a statistically smaller diurnal amplitude among women (0.43°C) versus men (0.55°C). Mallette et al. [28] also found an earlier bathyphase for women (at 4:48 AM) compared with men (at 6:04 AM) and also measured a much later

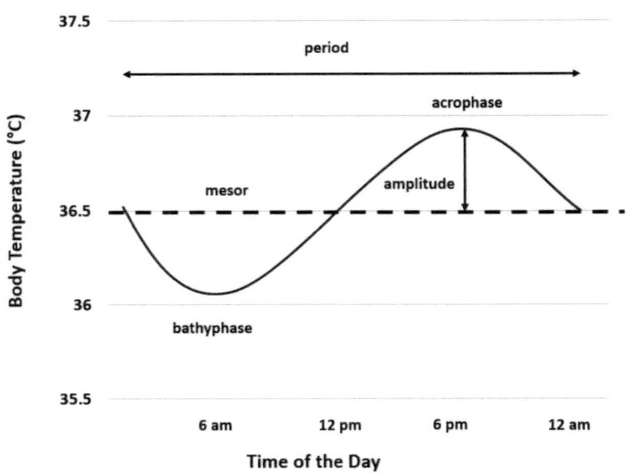

Figure 3.
Body temperature circadian rhythm schematic.

acrophase for women (at 10:49 PM) compared with men (at 8:49 PM). The authors of these studies hypothesized that the measured differences in the timing of acrophases and bathyphases could be related to the different timing of melatonin peak between the sexes. However, a highly controlled study by Gunn et al. [30] showed that although melatonin production and subsequently serum concentrations were higher in women, the circadian rhythm of melatonin, i.e., the timing of peak and trough, were statistically identical for both sexes. On the other hand, it was hypothesized that sex hormone-related differences could account for the lower diurnal change but not for the above detailed differences in acrophase and bathyphase timing [31, 32].

Further, age seems to be affecting the circadian rhythm as well. Czeisler et al. [29] showed that among healthy subjects the diurnal body temperature amplitude was significantly higher among younger individuals (average of 0.28°C) compared with older adults (average of 0.2°C). The authors proposed that there are age-related changes in the mammalian intrinsic pacemaker (the suprachiasmatic nucleus (SCN) in the hypothalamus) that could account for the smaller amplitudes among people and animals of advanced age. This is supported by the finding that other circadian rhythm indicators such as the sleep-wake cycle are also shorter in older people [33, 34]. Further, as humans age, the SCN decreases in size, likely due to age-related microvascular disease that leads to the overall shrinkage of the human brain with age, with the total number of SCN cells decreasing as well [35, 36]. Perhaps the most striking evidence stems from animal models using rodents, where the sleep-wake cycle period and the amplitude of the body temperature oscillation were shown to be directly proportional to the size of the remaining volume of the SCN in animals with partial lesions inflicted in that brain region [37, 38], with total loss of the circadian rhythm of body temperature upon complete surgical removal of the SCN [39]. However, it should be pointed out that traumatic brain injury in rats not involving the SCN specifically also had been shown to induce downregulation of circadian clock gene expression and associated animal behavioral changes [40], thus pointing to a more complex regulatory process of the mammalian circadian rhythm.

Although the complexity of body temperature regulation in man is great, ultimately a specific body temperature is the result of a balance between heat production via body metabolism and heat loss via processes such as heat radiation from and air convection at the body surface. Like we mentioned in the previous paragraph, the master pacemaker for all circadian cycles of the mammalian body, including body temperature, is believed to be located in the suprachiasmatic nucleus (SCN) of the hypothalamus, with abundant evidence thereof recently reviewed by Hastings et al. [41]. In a most simplistic description, body temperature information needs to be captured from the periphery, e.g., the extremities and the internal organs, then transported to the SCN, where it is processed, compared to the expected pre-set body temperature goal for the current location along the diurnal circadian cycle, then instructions for adjustments in heat production need to be sent from the SCN to the periphery and executed at the cellular level, with the ultimate result being a rise or fall in body temperature. To aid this temperature "normalization" process, there are also behavioral adaptations that animals exhibit such as seeking shade when the environment is too hot or moving to a warmer place when it is too cold. Certainly, the majority of modern humans have many more behavioral adaptations at their disposal compared with mammals living in the wild.

The specific mechanisms for some of these steps are well understood while others are still being investigated, with several recently published reviews available in the literature [17, 41, 42]. In mammals, including humans, temperature is sensed by TRP (transient receptor potential) family of ion channels [43–45]. The TRPs are expressed in sensory neurons throughout the body, with the biggest contributors to the signal being the skin, spinal cord, abdominal viscera, and the brain [46]. Different subtypes of TRPs are activated at different temperature thresholds [47] and the temperature information from the various sources is believed to be collected and processed by the SCN [48]. The SCN then communicates with the neurons in the preoptic area of the hypothalamus, which initiate the downstream signaling to achieve a "correction" in the organism's body temperature via the physiologic effectors that control thermogenesis, shivering, skin blood flow, and evaporative cooling as well as via thermoregulatory behaviors [49, 50]. The details regarding the various signaling cascades involved in the downstream signaling are still an area of active research. How the master pacemaker in the SCN operates is also being debated. There is some evidence pointing toward synchronization (a.k.a., entrainment) of the SCN by the ambient day-night lightening pattern [51–53]. Other studies provide evidence for hormonal regulation via melatonin feedback loops [54, 55] and via fluctuations in the serum serotonin levels [56, 57].

Regarding the circadian clock signaling mechanisms on the cellular level of multicellular organisms, these are being detailed in other chapters of this book. But briefly, in nearly all cells, including the SCN neurons, there is a clock-like mechanism in the form of an auto-regulatory transcriptional negative feedback loop as follows: The proteins CLOCK and BMAL1 (brain and muscle Arnt-like protein-1) form a dimer, which serves as a transcription factor and activates the transcription of the period and cryptochrome genes, which are then translated into the PER and CRY proteins. The PER and CRY proteins then interact with CLOCK and BMAL1, preventing them from further activating the period and cryptochrome genes' transcription. The CLOCK:BMAL1 transcription factor had been shown to also facilitate the expression of the clock-controlled genes (Ccgs), which are believed to control about 30% of the mammalian genome expression, thus controlling physiologic functions involved in metabolism, immunity, and many others [58]. To offer an example relevant to the circadian rhythm of body temperature, one of the downstream effects of this transcription loop involves the generation of oscillations in the mitochondrial oxidative capacity in mice via rhythmic changes of NAD+ biosynthesis [59]. These oscillations lead to changes in metabolic rate on the cellular level, which could potentially lead to a change in body temperature on the organismal level. All in all, at the current stage of scientific knowledge, the mechanisms that link the metabolic circadian rhythm at the cellular level to the circadian rhythm on the organismal level remain largely uncertain. What is curious however is the finding that even though an organism's body temperature diurnal cycling is governed by the circadian rhythm generated by the SCN, the diurnal temperature cycling itself is sufficient to sustain peripheral circadian clocks. This had been demonstrated by Brown et al. [60] in experiments where peripheral tissues from mammals were cultured *ex vivo*. The authors showed that by simulating the *in vivo* body temperature cycling inside the incubator, the tissues were able to maintain the proper circadian gene expression patterns. This points toward the existence of interdependence between the master clock in the SCN and body temperature. Beyond doubt, more research needs to be carried out before we can have a complete mechanistic picture for the maintenance of our body temperature. In parallel, knowledge regarding the clinical implications of disturbance in the body temperature diurnal rhythmicity had been accumulating and is explored in the next chapter section.

4. Fever, hypothermia, and other disruptions to the human body temperature circadian rhythm

Numerous studies had been carried out to demonstrate how disruption in the circadian rhythm of body temperature can affect human health. Perhaps the most extreme situations are those where fever or hypothermia completely obliterate the circadian rhythm balance. To better understand the clinical implications of these disruptions, we need to define fever and hypothermia. It had been known for a long time that a pyrogen (such as bacteria, viruses, toxins, and others) triggers "fever" by causing the release of prostaglandin E2, which acts on the preoptic area of the hypothalamus (a.k.a., the mammalian thermostat) to make it raise the temperature set point [61]. A higher temperature set-point results in a systemic body response attempting to raise the peripheral body temperature via active heat generation and by heat retention. Fever (pyrexia) in humans is associated with high inflammatory states such as sepsis and trauma [62]. Elevation of body temperature promotes the activation and trafficking of immune cells— in the case of T-lymphocytes, cell mobilization is achieved via a thermal sensory pathway involving alpha4 integrins and heat shock protein 90 [63]. On the other hand, hypothermia is a state of lower-than-normal hypothalamic setpoint. It occurs in settings such as severe debility due to illness leading to the inability to raise the body temperature; brain injury involving the preoptic area including age-related microvascular brain damage, stroke, and traumatic brain injury; congenital malformation of the preoptic area; seizure disorders, and likely others [64]. Hypothermia is associated with the inability to mount a strong inflammatory reaction and this is the reason why induced hypothermia had been used in some patients of cardiac arrest, where inflammation needs to be suppressed in order to allow time for the cardiac tissues to recover from the ischemic injury [65].

Deviations from normothermia among critically ill patients had been extensively studied. These deviations manifest in most such patients and appear to carry a prognostic value. For instance, a study by Sunden-Cullberg et al. [66] demonstrated that the ability among critically ill septic patients to mount fever while in the emergency department, i.e., before their admission to the ICU, was associated with lower in-hospital mortality and shorter hospital length of stay. On the other hand, Kiekkas et al. [67] showed that among the 239 ICU patients without cerebral damage such as stroke or neurosurgery in their study, fever was not associated with mortality but there was statistically significant increase in mortality with each 1°C increase in sustained maximal body temperature, indicating too much of a good thing (fever and the associated heightened immunity levels) can be harmful. Further, Peres Bota et al. [68] studied 439 ICU patients, not excluding any patients such as those with cerebral damage or those undergoing hypothermia protocols e.g., following cardiac arrest. These researchers found that both fever and hypothermia were associated with increased morbidity and mortality but those with hypothermia had a worse survival rate than the febrile patients. A potential confounding factor there was the fact that the hypothermic patients were significantly older compared with the patients with fever and it is common sense that older age is associate with less favorable clinical outcomes. In the case of patients with cerebral injury, studying 251 hospitalized subjects Schwartz et al. [69] demonstrated worse outcomes for patients with persistent fever and intracerebral hemorrhage, while Bao et al. [70] found similar results among their 355 patents with traumatic brain injury.

Regarding alterations in the body temperature circadian rhythms, these had been shown to occur in a variety of ways among the critically ill, including erratic acrophases, bathyphases, amplitudes, even complete abolishment of the cycling pattern [71–74]. Specifically, Tweedie et al. [71] showed that among the 15 intensive care unit (ICU) patients in their study, the acrophases varied by several hours from day to day both between patients and within the same individual patients over the study period of at least 8 ICU days per patient. Nuttall et al. [72] evaluated 149 ICU patients and reported that nearly all lacked a circadian rhythmicity of body temperature with the bathyphases distributed randomly throughout each 24-hour period. Paul et al. [73] studied 48 ICU patients and demonstrated major disturbance and often complete abolishment of the circadian rhythm as given by body temperature, melatonin and cortisol levels, blood pressure, heart rate, and spontaneous motor activity, all of which are known to be cycling with a 24-hour period in healthy individuals. Pina et al. [74] evaluated 8 patients managed in the burn ICU for 30 days and demonstrated the lack of circadian rhythm based on body temperature, melatonin, and cortisol levels for all patients during the entire hospitalization, although the authors noted a trend toward normalization of the body temperature diurnal cycle for some of the patients during the later stages of hospitalization. The latter two studies described above were prospective in design, thus providing more frequent data points, which may correspond to higher reliability but the overall conclusion based on all research findings is that critical illness is associated with major disturbance in the circadian rhythm of human body temperature.

The clinical prognostication value of human body temperature circadian rhythm variations is remarkable as well. Blume et al. [75] demonstrated that among their 18 patients with severe brain injury leading to loss of consciousness, preservation of the body temperature diurnal cycling was associated with increased chance for recovering from their comatose state. Further, Tweedie et al. [71] found that among their 15 ICU patients, there was a bigger circadian rhythm amplitude during periods of unconsciousness compared with when patients were conscious and the amplitudes were also bigger among the patients who died compared to those who survived. In a larger study of 248 patients with severe trauma admitted to the ICU and excluding any patients who had undergone targeted hypothermia protocol following cardiac arrest, Culver et al. [76] found that disruption in the body temperature circadian rhythm with mesor <36.9°C and amplitude >0.6°C were associated with higher 28-day-all-cause mortality. They also showed that the association was more pronounced among patients with head trauma compared with those with non-head trauma. Among the general ICU patient population comprising of 21 patients, Gazendam et al. [77] documented an acrophase shift in 81% of the studied patients and also found that the severity of illness, as given by the APACHE III (Acute Physiology and Chronic Health Evaluation) score, was predictive of the magnitude of circadian misplacement. Importantly, it was demonstrated by Drewry et al. [78] how in the ICU setting one can monitor the diurnal body temperature oscillations and look for specific disruptions in the rhythm that had been associated with the early development of sepsis, thus providing an early sepsis warning before the traditional sepsis criterial are met, which in turn would allow for an earlier intervention with antibiotics. Given all the clinical data, it is fair to conclude that disruption of the circadian rhythm and deviation from normothermia among the critically ill likely facilitates a mal-adaptive and hyperactive (in the case of fever) or hypoactive (in the case of hypothermia) inflammatory responses that can lead to organismal failure and death.

The importance of the circadian rhythm has also been demonstrated in non-critically ill hospitalized patients. For instance, our group [79] found that among the 16,245 hospitalized patients included in the study, the circadian rhythm was disrupted in 80%. Further, we reported an age-dependent shift in the circadian pattern, with the body temperature bathyphase of older people shifted to 12 pm in the afternoon (compared with 8 am for young adults) but with the acrophase among the old remaining at 8 pm, similar to the younger patient cohort. (**Figure 4**, adopted with modifications and permission from Geneva et al. [79]). After considering other theories, we had concluded that the most likely explanation for the circadian body temperature disruption during hospitalization was the disturbance in the patients' day-night light cycles caused by frequent awaking at night for procedures, vital signs measurements, and the associated exposure to light during the night. Several other studies with human subjects have also supported the role of diurnal light levels in resetting the human circadian clock [80–84]. Similar to the ICU patients, body temperature measurements from non-critically ill patients appear to carry prognostic value as demonstrated by Obermeyer et al. [11]. The authors studied the body temperature of over 35,000 hospitalized patients, who were not diagnosed with infection and did not receive antibiotics; they showed that after adjustment for age and comorbidities that could affect body temperature (e.g., hypothyroidism is associated with lower body temperature, active cancer is associated with higher body temperature), there was correlation between deviation from the expected normothermia range and the one-year mortality.

On the outpatient basis, the disruption of the natural circadian rhythm emerged as an important player in disease pathogenesis via epidemiologic studies in the 1990s that linked it to the development of cancers among night shift workers. Specifically, higher levels of breast cancer were noted among Norwegian radio and telegraph operators [85]. Further research also demonstrated increased incidence of colorectal and prostate cancers as well as metabolic and gastrointestinal disorders among people working night shifts [86–88]. In this population of workers, various circadian rhythm

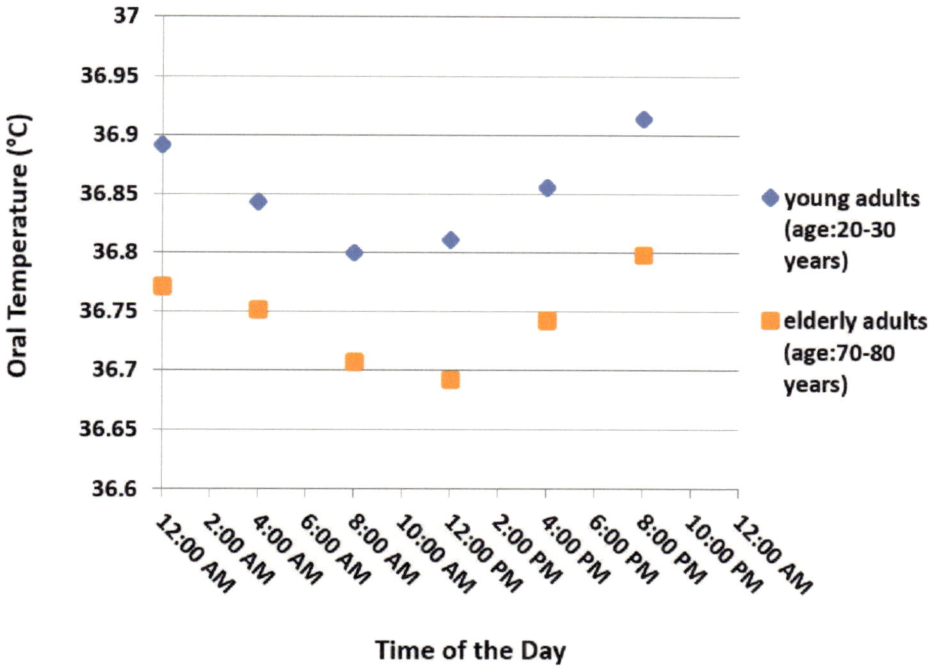

Figure 4.
Diurnal body temperature variation of hospitalized patients classified by age. Adapted with modifications and with permission from Geneva et al. [79] ***Figure 2A****.*

markers such as melatonin and cortisol blood levels as well as the diurnal cycling of body temperature were shown to be disturbed [89–92]. The situation was further aggravated by the realization that these circadian abnormalities persist for years after retirement from night shift work jobs [92, 93]. It should be mentioned that not all research had been supportive of these associations; namely a recent meta-analysis by Dun et al. [94] evaluated 57 observational studies and concluded that there was no association between any exposure to night shift work during subjects' lifetime and increased risk for several common solid cancers, albeit there were several major caveats regarding the data heterogeneity. Notwithstanding the meta-analysis results, researchers theorized that light exposure at night facilitates the carcinogenesis via disruption of the natural melatonin cycle in humans. Melatonin is believed to have a second function, in addition to neuro-hormonal signaling, where it acts as a scavenger of reactive oxygen species [95]. As melatonin production occurs at night and it is suppressed by light, exposure to light during night shift-work leads to less melatonin production and supposedly accumulation of oxygen radicals, which constitute a known risk for the development of malignancies [96]. In support of this theory, it was demonstrated that women with complete blindness (no light perception) had significantly lower prevalence of breast cancer compared with blind women with preserved light perception [97]. Research with mice had provided more specific evidence, where melatonin knockout animals prone to breast cancer development (p53(R270H/+)WAPCre conditional mutant mice) suffer from faster tumor growth in shift work simulation experiments as compared to animals with the same breast cancer predisposition but with normal melatonin production [98]. Over the years, sufficient evidence had accumulated from epidemiological studies and animal model research to prompt the Agency for Research on Cancer to classify shift work involving circadian rhythm disruption as likely carcinogenic [99]. This is a good place to point out that in the current era of technological advance, a large portion of Earth's population is living in conditions akin to night shift workers' due to the extensive use of digital devices (cell phones, tablets, TV, etc.) late into the night, thus leading to the so called social jetlag and likely circadian misalignment [100, 101].

It is well established that a weakened immune system is a predisposition to the growth of malignancies, with cancer immunotherapy currently being a hot area of research [102]. As such, the above-described associations between circadian rhythm disruption and cancer may stem from the effect of circadian rhythm abnormality on the immune system, which was previously reviewed by Logan et al. [103], Comas et al. [104], and Coiffard et al. [105]. While most research had been done in animal models, human studies did show that disruption of the circadian rhythm (induced with a sleep desynchronization protocol) negatively affects the human transcriptome [106]. Namely, the authors found a reduction in the normal diurnally-guided rhythmic transcription from a baseline of 6.4% to 1.0%. Many of the genes affected by this transcription reduction are known to play important roles in immune pathways, including cytokine and NFκB signaling [106, 107]. The effect of the circadian rhythmicity on one's immunity could also explain the observation from mice animal models where disease severity was higher if a pulmonary infection with Streptococcus *pneumoniae* was induced during the resting phase of the animals (when their body temperature is lower) compared with infecting them during their active phase (when their body temperature is higher) [108].

In addition to associations with cancer and immunologic dysfunction, night shift-work-related circadian rhythm disturbance had been linked to cardiovascular risk factors such as decrease in insulin sensitivity and decrease in leptin (the satiety hormone) blood levels [109–114]. Other published reports have demonstrated links to cognitive and psychiatric disorders as reviewed by Karatsoreos et al. [115]. These include decreased reaction time, increased error rate, and temporal lobe atrophy among flight attendants serving on frequent trans-Atlantic flights leading to jet-lag-induced circadian rhythm desynchronization [116]; correlation between the intensity of major depression attacks with the size of delays in the circadian pacemaker as regards the timing of sleep onset [117]; reduction in the self-reported mood and well-being level among healthy volunteers who were subjected to a sleep-wake circadian rhythm disruption experimental protocol [118]. Even the gut microbiota was shown to be altered upon disruption of the circadian rhythm based on light-dark cycling in animal models using mice [119] and Drosophila [120]. It should be noted that the experimental findings detailed in this paragraph do not directly link disruption in the body temperature circadian rhythm to the identified behavioral or physical health conditions and deficits. Still, body temperature is the most easily measured indicator of circadian rhythm preservation or disruption. As such, its application in the design of experimental paradigms and tests for the effects of medical interventions is expected to be of great benefit to future research, which is the focus of the next chapter section.

5. Future directions in body temperature and chronotherapy research

The last two centuries saw a great advancement in our knowledge of the circadian rhythm of living organisms. Yet, much remains to be discovered as relates to both molecular pathways and clinical applications to improve human health. In particular, at the current stage of scientific knowledge, the mechanism that links the circadian rhythm at the cellular level to the circadian rhythm of body temperature on the organismal level remains unknown. Also, there is a significant heterogeneity among human studies, thus making the confirmation of specific associations between disruption in the circadian rhythm and human disease challenging. Further, the clinical interventions currently in use are at best crude and not optimized to reach their full potential. One example is the use of a melatonin pill in the evening to fight insomnia, where research regarding the dose or time of intake remains inconclusive and the effects are modest, as detailed in a metanalysis by Ferracioli-Oda et al. [121]. Another example would be the use of very bright light (7000 to 12,000 lux with the associated possible light damage to the retina) instead of the ordinary 150 lux during night shifts, which was shown to lead to circadian rhythm adaptation to shift work after 4 days of treatment as evidenced by the delay in the body temperature nadir from 3:30 AM to 2:50 PM and improvement in cognitive performance and alertness among healthy volunteers [122]. It should also be pointed out that a big portion of the existing knowledge stems from animal model research and needs validation in humans before wide-spread application in clinical settings could be attempted. What is perhaps most relevant to this book chapter is the fact that the vast majority of circadian rhythm research uses the day-night wake-sleep pattern and measurements of serum biomarkers such as melatonin. Measuring body temperature as the human circadian rhythm marker would be a much less resource-heavy and less invasive approach in research designs. Thanks to the recent advances in electronics, the monitoring of human body temperature can be done at high frequency (collecting several measurements per minute) using relatively inexpensive equipment for data collection with wearable devices that allow for research to be carried out even outside hospitals and research centers. An important requirement for all research involving body temperature would be accurate temperature measurement via careful device calibration and by ensuring the temperature collection site is not significantly influenced by environmental temperature fluctuations or alternatively devising an algorithm to correct for any external variables.

Many of the experiments that so far involved animal models can be repeated in humans using body temperature as the main circadian rhythm measure. For instance, using the Gibbs et al. encouraging pre-clinical results regarding bacterial infections in mice [108], a human challenge model experimental protocol could be built as follows. One could inflict skin cuts on one arm of healthy volunteers during the day (near the body temperature acrophase) and on the other arm during the night (near the body temperature bathyphase). Then, one would quantify the inflammatory response and the evolution of the infection of each cut, where each person serves as their own internal control. If there is significant difference in the infection severity and healing times akin to the difference observed in mice, then this experiment could inform the timing of surgical procedures based on each patient's specific circadian rhythm. Such an approach would constitute another step toward personalized medicine.

As detailed earlier in this chapter, disruption in the body temperature diurnal cycling pattern can be used as a predictor of events such as early sepsis, it can serve as a predictor of patient outcome among the critically ill, it can monitor the success (or lack thereof) of circadian adaptation in night shift workers, and the list goes on. But if any of these applications are to be used as standard of care tools, we would need well-controlled multi-institutional studies to validate the potential early warning system and clinical prediction models. In order to improve model validity, data from body temperature oscillations will likely have to be combined with other types of information such as the non-temperature vital signs, comorbidities, age, race, environmental specifications such as level of lightning, etc. Similar considerations apply to interventional studies such as light therapy to re-establish the circadian rhythm in night shift workers and people with psychiatric illnesses. Research aiming to identify the most optimal time along the circadian cycle for chemotherapy [123] or antibiotics [124] delivery constitutes yet another promising avenue open for exploration. Given the complexity of the involved models, the field of chronotherapy could prove an opportunity for the application of artificial intelligence to optimize the various model variables.

In conclusion, ours are exciting times for circadian rhythm research and the circadian rhythm of human body temperature provides an easily accessible tool for the development of clinically relevant applications.

Author details

Ivayla I. Geneva
Crouse Hospital, Syracuse, NY, USA

*Address all correspondence to: geneva.ivayla@gmail.com

References

[1] Boeck B. Diagnose im Alten Mesopotamien. Ueberlegungen zu Graenzen und Moeglichkeiten der Interpretation keilschriftlicher diagnostischer Texte. Orientalistische Literaturzeitung. 2009;**104**(4-5):382-398

[2] Geller MJ. West meets east: Early Greek and Babylonian diagnosis. In: Horstmanshoff FJ, Stol M, editors. Magic and Rationality in Acient near Eastern and Graeco-Roman Medicine. Leiden-Boston: Brill; 2004

[3] Heessel N. Babylonisch-assyrische Diagnostik. Muenster: Ugarit-Verlag; 2000

[4] Heessel N. Reading and interpreting medical cuneiform texts-methods and problems. Le Journal des Medecines Cuneiformed. 2004;**3**:6-7

[5] Wunderlich CRA, Das Verhalten der Eigenwaerme in Krankheiten. Leipzig: Verlag von Otto Wigand; 1868

[6] Geneva II et al. Normal body temperature: A systematic review. Open Forum Infectious Diseases. 2019;**6**(4):ofz032

[7] Mackowiak PA, Wasserman SS, Levine MM. A critical appraisal of 98.6 degrees F, the upper limit of the normal body temperature, and other legacies of Carl Reinhold august Wunderlich. JAMA. 1992;**268**(12):1578-1580

[8] Chamberlain JM et al. Determination of normal ear temperature with an infrared emission detection thermometer. Annals of Emergency Medicine. 1995;**25**(1):15-20

[9] Horvath SM, Menduke H, Piersol GM. Oral and rectal temperatures of man. Journal of the American Medical Association. 1950;**144**(18):1562-1565

[10] Harding C et al. The daily, weekly, and seasonal cycles of body temperature analyzed at large scale. Chronobiology International. 2019;**36**(12):1646-1657

[11] Obermeyer Z, Samra JK, Mullainathan S. Individual differences in normal body temperature: Longitudinal big data analysis of patient records. BMJ. 2017;**359**:j5468

[12] Diamond A et al. One size does not fit all: Assuming the same normal body temperature for everyone is not justified. PLoS One. 2021;**16**(2):e0245257

[13] Corsi AJSM, Lupone C, Geneva II. 1022. The role of baseline body temperature in neutropenic fever. Open Forum Infectious Diseases. 2022;**9**:863

[14] Protsiv M et al. Decreasing human body temperature in the United States since the industrial revolution. eLife. 2020;**9**:e49555

[15] Frazer JS et al. Variability in body temperature in healthy adults and in patients receiving chemotherapy: Prospective observational cohort study. Journal of Medical Engineering & Technology. 2019;**43**(5):323-333

[16] Refinetti R. The circadian rhythm of body temperature. Front Bioscience (Landmark Ed). 2010;**15**:564-594

[17] Refinetti R. Circadian rhythmicity of body temperature and metabolism. Temperature (Austin). 2020;**7**(4):321-362

[18] Rijo-Ferreira F, Takahashi JS, Figueiredo LM. Circadian rhythms

in parasites. PLoS Pathogens. 2017;**13**(10):e1006590

[19] Bhadra U et al. Evolution of circadian rhythms: From bacteria to human. Sleep Medicine. 2017;**35**:49-61

[20] Dibner C, Schibler U, Albrecht U. The mammalian circadian timing system: Organization and coordination of central and peripheral clocks. Annual Review of Physiology. 2010;**72**:517-549

[21] Suvorov NB et al. High precision human skin temperature fluctuations measuring instrument. Sensors (Basel). 2021;**21**(12):4101

[22] Flora C et al. High-frequency temperature monitoring for early detection of febrile adverse events in patients with cancer. Cancer Cell. 2021;**39**(9):1167-1168

[23] Davy J. Researches Physiological and Anatomical. London: Smith, Elder and Co.; 1839

[24] Ogle W. On the diurnal variations of the temperature of the human body in health. St George's Hosp Rep. 1866;**1**:221-245

[25] Minors DS, Waterhouse JM. Circadian Rhythms and the Human. Bristol, Great Britain: Wright . PSG; 1981

[26] Baker FC et al. Sleep and 24 hour body temperatures: A comparison in young men, naturally cycling women and women taking hormonal contraceptives. The Journal of Physiology. 2001;**530**(Pt 3):565-574

[27] Cain SW et al. Sex differences in phase angle of entrainment and melatonin amplitude in humans. Journal of Biological Rhythms. 2010;**25**(4):288-296

[28] Mellette HC et al. Diurnal variations in body temperatures. Journal of Applied Physiology. 1951;**3**(11):665-675

[29] Czeisler CA et al. Association of sleep-wake habits in older people with changes in output of circadian pacemaker. Lancet. 1992;**340**(8825):933-936

[30] Gunn PJ et al. Sex differences in the circadian profiles of melatonin and cortisol in plasma and urine matrices under constant routine conditions. Chronobiology International. 2016;**33**(1):39-50

[31] Mortola JP. Gender and the circadian pattern of body temperature in normoxia and hypoxia. Respiratory Physiology & Neurobiology. 2017;**245**:4-12

[32] Nakayama K et al. Circadian changes in body temperature during the menstrual cycle of healthy adult females and patients suffering from premenstrual syndrome. International Journal of Clinical Pharmacology Research. 1997;**17**(4):155-164

[33] Weitzman ED et al. Chronobiology of aging: Temperature, sleep-wake rhythms and entrainment. Neurobiology of Aging. 1982;**3**(4):299-309

[34] Czeisler CA et al. Bright light resets the human circadian pacemaker independent of the timing of the sleep-wake cycle. Science. 1986;**233**(4764):667-671

[35] Hofman MA et al. Morphometric analysis of the suprachiasmatic and paraventricular nuclei in the human brain: Sex differences and age-dependent changes. Journal of Anatomy. 1988;**160**:127-143

[36] Swaab DF, Fliers E, Partiman TS. The suprachiasmatic nucleus of the

human brain in relation to sex, age and senile dementia. Brain Research. 1985;**342**(1):37-44

[37] Abe K et al. Effects of destruction of the suprachiasmatic nuclei on the circadian rhythms in plasma corticosterone, body temperature, feeding and plasma thyrotropin. Neuroendocrinology. 1979;**29**(2):119-131

[38] Davis FC, Gorski RA. Unilateral lesions of the hamster suprachiasmatic nuclei: Evidence for redundant control of circadian rhythms. Journal of Comparative Physiology. 1984;**154**:221-232

[39] Ruby NF et al. The suprachiasmatic nucleus is essential for circadian body temperature rhythms in hibernating ground squirrels. The Journal of Neuroscience. 2002;**22**(1):357-364

[40] Boone DR et al. Traumatic brain injury-induced dysregulation of the circadian clock. PLoS One. 2012;7(10):e46204

[41] Hastings MH, Maywood ES, Brancaccio M. Generation of circadian rhythms in the suprachiasmatic nucleus. Nature Reviews. Neuroscience. 2018;**19**(8):453-469

[42] Koch CE et al. Interaction between circadian rhythms and stress. Neurobiology of Stress. 2017;**6**:57-67

[43] Wang H, Siemens J. TRP ion channels in thermosensation, thermoregulation and metabolism. Temperature (Austin). 2015;**2**(2):178-187

[44] Caterina MJ. Transient receptor potential ion channels as participants in thermosensation and thermoregulation. American Journal of Physiology. Regulatory, Integrative and Comparative Physiology. 2007;**292**(1):R64-R76

[45] Yue WWS et al. TRPV1 drugs alter core body temperature via central projections of primary afferent sensory neurons. eLife. 2022;**11**:e80139

[46] Cabanac M. Temperature regulation. Annual Review of Physiology. 1975;**37**:415-439

[47] Lezama-Garcia K et al. Transient receptor potential (TRP) and thermoregulation in animals: Structural biology and neurophysiological aspects. Animals (Basel). 2022;**12**(1):106

[48] Poletini MO et al. TRP channels: A missing bond in the entrainment mechanism of peripheral clocks throughout evolution. Temperature (Austin). 2015;**2**(4):522-534

[49] Rothhaas R, Chung S. Role of the preoptic area in sleep and thermoregulation. Frontiers in Neuroscience. 2021;**15**:664781

[50] Tan CL, Knight ZA. Regulation of body temperature by the nervous system. Neuron. 2018;**98**(1):31-48

[51] Mazuski C et al. Entrainment of circadian rhythms depends on firing rates and neuropeptide release of VIP SCN neurons. Neuron. 2018;**99**(3):555-563 e5

[52] Ding JM et al. Resetting the biological clock: Mediation of nocturnal CREB phosphorylation via light, glutamate, and nitric oxide. The Journal of Neuroscience. 1997;**17**(2):667-675

[53] Wright KP Jr et al. Entrainment of the human circadian clock to the natural light-dark cycle. Current Biology. 2013;**23**(16):1554-1558

[54] Waly NE, Hallworth R. Circadian pattern of melatonin MT1 and MT2 receptor localization in the rat Suprachiasmatic nucleus. Journal of Circadian Rhythms. 2015;**13**:1

[55] Cajochen C, Krauchi K, Wirz-Justice A. Role of melatonin in the regulation of human circadian rhythms and sleep. Journal of Neuroendocrinology. 2003;**15**(4):432-437

[56] Meyer-Bernstein EL, Morin LP. Differential serotonergic innervation of the suprachiasmatic nucleus and the intergeniculate leaflet and its role in circadian rhythm modulation. The Journal of Neuroscience. 1996;**16**(6):2097-2111

[57] Miyamoto H et al. Serotonergic integration of circadian clock and ultradian sleep-wake cycles. The Journal of Neuroscience. 2012;**32**(42):14794-14803

[58] Tognini P et al. Distinct circadian signatures in liver and gut clocks revealed by ketogenic diet. Cell Metabolism. 2017;**26**(3):523-538 e5

[59] Peek CB et al. Circadian clock NAD+ cycle drives mitochondrial oxidative metabolism in mice. Science. 2013;**342**(6158):1243417

[60] Brown SA et al. Rhythms of mammalian body temperature can sustain peripheral circadian clocks. Current Biology. 2002;**12**(18):1574-1583

[61] Scammell TE et al. Ventromedial preoptic prostaglandin E2 activates fever-producing autonomic pathways. The Journal of Neuroscience. 1996;**16**(19):6246-6254

[62] Evans SS, Repasky EA, Fisher DT. Fever and the thermal regulation of immunity: The immune system feels the heat. Nature Reviews. Immunology. 2015;**15**(6):335-349

[63] Lin C et al. Fever promotes T lymphocyte trafficking via a thermal sensory pathway involving heat shock protein 90 and alpha4 Integrins. Immunity. 2019;**50**(1):137-151 e6

[64] Blondin NA. Diagnosis and management of periodic hypothermia. Neurological Clinical Practice. 2014;**4**(1):26-33

[65] Nolan JP et al. Therapeutic hypothermia after cardiac arrest: An advisory statement by the advanced life support task force of the international liaison committee on resuscitation. Circulation. 2003;**108**(1):118-121

[66] Sunden-Cullberg J et al. Fever in the emergency department predicts survival of patients with severe sepsis and septic shock admitted to the ICU. Critical Care Medicine. 2017;**45**(4):591-599

[67] Kiekkas P et al. Peak body temperature predicts mortality in critically ill patients without cerebral damage. Heart & Lung. 2010;**39**(3):208-216

[68] Peres Bota D et al. Body temperature alterations in the critically ill. Intensive Care Medicine. 2004;**30**(5):811-816

[69] Schwarz S et al. Incidence and prognostic significance of fever following intracerebral hemorrhage. Neurology. 2000;**54**(2):354-361

[70] Bao L et al. Fever burden is an independent predictor for prognosis of traumatic brain injury. PLoS One. 2014;**9**(3):e90956

[71] Tweedie IE et al. Retrospective study of temperature rhythms of intensive care patients. Critical Care Medicine. 1989;**17**(11):1159-1165

[72] Nuttall GA, Kumar M, Murray MJ. No difference exists in the alteration

of circadian rhythm between patients with and without intensive care unit psychosis. Critical Care Medicine. 1998;**26**(8):1351-1355

[73] Paul T, Lemmer B. Disturbance of circadian rhythms in analgosedated intensive care unit patients with and without craniocerebral injury. Chronobiology International. 2007;**24**(1):45-61

[74] Pina G et al. Long-term alteration of daily melatonin, 6-sulfatoxymelatonin, cortisol, and temperature profiles in burn patients: A preliminary report. Chronobiology International. 2010;**27**(2):378-392

[75] Blume C et al. Significance of circadian rhythms in severely brain-injured patients: A clue to consciousness? Neurology. 2017;**88**(20):1933-1941

[76] Culver A et al. Circadian disruption of core body temperature in trauma patients: A single-center retrospective observational study. Journal of Intensive Care. 2020;**8**:4

[77] Gazendam JAC et al. Altered circadian rhythmicity in patients in the ICU. Chest. 2013;**144**(2):483-489

[78] Drewry AM et al. Body temperature patterns as a predictor of hospital-acquired sepsis in afebrile adult intensive care unit patients: A case-control study. Critical Care. 2013;**17**(5):R200

[79] Geneva, II and W. Javaid, Disruption of the body temperature circadian rhythm in hospitalized patients. The American Journal of the Medical Sciences, 2021. 362(6): p. 578-585.

[80] Boivin DB et al. Dose-response relationships for resetting of human circadian clock by light. Nature. 1996;**379**(6565):540-542

[81] Czeisler CA et al. Stability, precision, and near-24-hour period of the human circadian pacemaker. Science. 1999;**284**(5423):2177-2181

[82] Klerman EB et al. Simulations of light effects on the human circadian pacemaker: Implications for assessment of intrinsic period. The American Journal of Physiology. 1996;**270**(1 Pt 2): R271-R282

[83] Phillips AJK et al. High sensitivity and interindividual variability in the response of the human circadian system to evening light. Proceedings of the National Academy of Sciences of the United States of America. 2019;**116**(24):12019-12024

[84] Zeitzer JM et al. Sensitivity of the human circadian pacemaker to nocturnal light: Melatonin phase resetting and suppression. The Journal of Physiology. 2000;**526**(Pt 3):695-702

[85] Tynes T et al. Incidence of breast cancer in Norwegian female radio and telegraph operators. Cancer Causes & Control. 1996;**7**(2):197-204

[86] Knutsson A. Health disorders of shift workers. Occupational Medicine (London). 2003;**53**(2):103-108

[87] Schernhammer ES et al. Night-shift work and risk of colorectal cancer in the nurses' health study. Journal of the National Cancer Institute. 2003;**95**(11):825-828

[88] Sigurdardottir LG et al. Circadian disruption, sleep loss, and prostate cancer risk: A systematic review of epidemiologic studies. Cancer Epidemiology, Biomarkers & Prevention. 2012;**21**(7):1002-1011

[89] Brum MCB et al. Effect of night-shift work on cortisol circadian rhythm

and melatonin levels. Sleep Science. 2022;**15**(2):143-148

[90] Li J et al. Impact of shift work on the diurnal cortisol rhythm: A one-year longitudinal study in junior physicians. Journal of Occupational Medicine and Toxicology. 2018;**13**:23

[91] Sack RL, Blood ML, Lewy AJ. Melatonin rhythms in night shift workers. Sleep. 1992;**15**(5):434-441

[92] Jang TW et al. Circadian rhythm of wrist temperature among shift Workers in South Korea: A prospective observational study. International Journal of Environmental Research and Public Health. 2017;**14**(10):1109

[93] Monk TH et al. Polysomnographic sleep and circadian temperature rhythms as a function of prior shift work exposure in retired seniors. Healthy Aging Clinical Care Elder. 2013;**2013**(5):9-19

[94] Dun A et al. Association between night-shift work and cancer risk: Updated systematic review and meta-analysis. Frontiers in Oncology. 2020;**10**:1006

[95] Zang LY et al. Scavenging of reactive oxygen species by melatonin. Biochimica et Biophysica Acta. 1998;**1425**(3):469-477

[96] Liou GY, Storz P. Reactive oxygen species in cancer. Free Radical Research. 2010;**44**(5):479-496

[97] Flynn-Evans EE et al. Total visual blindness is protective against breast cancer. Cancer Causes & Control. 2009;**20**(9):1753-1756

[98] Van Dycke KC et al. Chronically alternating light cycles increase breast cancer risk in mice. Current Biology. 2015;**25**(14):1932-1937

[99] Hansen J. Light at night, shiftwork, and breast cancer risk. Journal of the National Cancer Institute. 2001;**93**(20):1513-1515

[100] Roenneberg T, Merrow M. The circadian clock and human health. Current Biology. 2016;**26**(10):R432-R443

[101] Wittmann M et al. Social jetlag: Misalignment of biological and social time. Chronobiology International. 2006;**23**(1-2):497-509

[102] Hiam-Galvez KJ, Allen BM, Spitzer MH. Systemic immunity in cancer. Nature Reviews. Cancer. 2021;**21**(6):345-359

[103] Logan RW, Sarkar DK. Circadian nature of immune function. Molecular and Cellular Endocrinology. 2012;**349**(1):82-90

[104] Comas M et al. A circadian based inflammatory response – Implications for respiratory disease and treatment. Sleep Science and Practice. 2017;**1**(1):18

[105] Coiffard B et al. A tangled threesome: Circadian rhythm, body temperature variations, and the immune system. Biology (Basel). 2021;**10**(1):65

[106] Archer SN et al. Mistimed sleep disrupts circadian regulation of the human transcriptome. Proceedings of the National Academy of Sciences of the United States of America. 2014;**111**(6):E682-E691

[107] Moller-Levet CS et al. Effects of insufficient sleep on circadian rhythmicity and expression amplitude of the human blood transcriptome. Proceedings of the National Academy of Sciences of the United States of America. 2013;**110**(12):E1132-E1141

[108] Gibbs J et al. An epithelial circadian clock controls pulmonary inflammation

and glucocorticoid action. Nature Medicine. 2014;**20**(8):919-926

[109] Reutrakul S, Knutson KL. Consequences of circadian disruption on Cardiometabolic health. Sleep Medicine Clinics. 2015;**10**(4):455-468

[110] Buxton OM et al. Adverse metabolic consequences in humans of prolonged sleep restriction combined with circadian disruption. Science Translational Medicine. 2012;**4**(129):129ra43

[111] Scheer FA et al. Adverse metabolic and cardiovascular consequences of circadian misalignment. Proceedings of the National Academy of Sciences of the United States of America. 2009;**106**(11):4453-4458

[112] Leproult R, Holmback U, Van Cauter E. Circadian misalignment augments markers of insulin resistance and inflammation, independently of sleep loss. Diabetes. 2014;**63**(6):1860-1869

[113] McHill AW et al. Impact of circadian misalignment on energy metabolism during simulated nightshift work. Proceedings of the National Academy of Sciences of the United States of America. 2014;**111**(48):17302-17307

[114] Morris CJ et al. Endogenous circadian system and circadian misalignment impact glucose tolerance via separate mechanisms in humans. Proceedings of the National Academy of Sciences of the United States of America. 2015;**112**(17):E2225-E2234

[115] Karatsoreos IN. Links between circadian rhythms and psychiatric disease. Frontiers in Behavioral Neuroscience. 2014;**8**:162

[116] Cho K. Chronic 'jet lag' produces temporal lobe atrophy and spatial cognitive deficits. Nature Neuroscience. 2001;**4**(6):567-568

[117] Emens J et al. Circadian misalignment in major depressive disorder. Psychiatry Research. 2009;**168**(3):259-261

[118] Chellappa SL, Morris CJ, Scheer F. Circadian misalignment increases mood vulnerability in simulated shift work. Scientific Reports. 2020;**10**(1):18614

[119] Liang X, Bushman FD, FitzGerald GA. Rhythmicity of the intestinal microbiota is regulated by gender and the host circadian clock. Proceedings of the National Academy of Sciences of the United States of America. 2015;**112**(33):10479-10484

[120] Zhang Y et al. The microbiome stabilizes circadian rhythms in the gut. Proceedings of the National Academy of Sciences of the United States of America. 2023;**120**(5):e2217532120

[121] Ferracioli-Oda E, Qawasmi A, Bloch MH. Meta-analysis: Melatonin for the treatment of primary sleep disorders. PLoS One. 2013;**8**(5):e63773

[122] Czeisler CA et al. Exposure to bright light and darkness to treat physiologic maladaptation to night work. The New England Journal of Medicine. 1990;**322**(18):1253-1259

[123] Levi F et al. Circadian timing in cancer treatments. Annual Review of Pharmacology and Toxicology. 2010;**50**:377-421

[124] Smolensky MH et al. Circadian disruption: New clinical perspective of disease pathology and basis for chronotherapeutic intervention. Chronobiology International. 2016;**33**(8):1101-1119

Chapter 9

Presepsin as a Diagnostic and Prognostic Biomarker in Sepsis

Sanja Stankovic

Abstract

Sepsis is defined as a life-threatening condition with organ failure, caused by an inadequate response of the host to the infection. It is a public health and economic problem worldwide. Early and accurate diagnosis of sepsis and timely inclusion of appropriate therapy are important for the outcome of the treatment of patients with sepsis. Sepsis biomarkers may provide information to achieve an early diagnosis, and predict prognosis and therapeutic response. Today, the literature lists more than 250 different biomarkers related to sepsis. However, stronger clinical evidence of clinical usefulness has emerged only for a few biomarkers from many published studies and meta-analyses. Among them, presepsin (sCD14-ST) appears to be one of the most promising biomarkers of sepsis in daily clinical practice. This chapter highlights the utility of presepsin as a diagnostic and prognostic biomarker of sepsis both in adult and pediatric patients.

Keywords: biomarker, diagnosis, infections, presepsin, prognosis, sepsis

1. Introduction

Sepsis is recognized as a global health problem worldwide and an important public health issue with considerable economic consequences. Sepsis can be the clinical manifestation of infections acquired both in the community setting and in health care facilities. Third International Consensus Definitions for Sepsis and Septic Shock (Sepsis-3) from 2016 defines sepsis as "life-threatening organ dysfunction caused by a dysregulated host response to infection." This definition emphasizes the central pathogenetic role of the non-homeostatic host response to microorganisms rather than the infection *per se* [1]. Organ dysfunction was described using scoring systems such as the Sequential (Sepsis-related) Organ Failure Assessment score (SOFA score). A SOFA score ≥ 2 points were set as a criterion for more rapid identifying patients with sepsis in intensive care units (ICU). Patients with a SOFA score of 2 or more had an overall mortality risk of approximately 10% in a general hospital population with suspected infection. Sepsis-3 has also introduced a new simpler score, called the quick Sequential Organ Failure Assessment (qSOFA) for use in non-ICU settings, to identify septic patients in out-of-hospital, emergency department, or general hospital ward setting. The qSOFA consists of three variables: respiratory rate ≥ 22 breaths per min, systolic blood pressure ≤ 100 mmHg, and altered mentation. A qSOFA score ≥ 2 was found to be significantly predictive of increased all-cause mortality in patients outside of the

IntechOpen

ICU. According to Sepsis-3 definition, septic shock was defined as a subset of sepsis in which underlying circulatory and metabolic abnormalities are profound enough to substantially increase mortality. Patients with septic shock can be clinically identified by a vasopressor requirement to maintain a mean arterial pressure of 65 mm Hg or greater and serum lactate level greater than 2 mmol/l (>18 mg/dl) in the absence of hypovolemia. This combination is associated with hospital mortality rates greater than 40% [1].

Neonatal sepsis is a systemic condition of bacterial, viral, or fungal (yeast) origin that is associated with hemodynamic changes and other clinical manifestations and results in substantial morbidity and mortality. The symptoms are variable and nonspecific. Based on the onset neonatal sepsis could be classified into two types: (a) early-onset sepsis (EOS), which manifests as respiratory distress within 72 h of birth, and is mainly due to bacteria acquired before and/or during delivery (maternal-fetal infection); (b) late-onset sepsis (LOS), which manifests as septicemia after 72 h of birth and is due to bacteria acquired after delivery like nosocomial ones (community or hospital-acquired), and affects preterm and very-low-birth-weight neonates in particular [2].

The global burden of sepsis is difficult to ascertain. A meta-analysis of studies on adults admitted to hospitals from seven high-income countries suggested global estimates of 31.5 million sepsis (19.4 million severe sepsis cases), and 5.3 million sepsis-related deaths annually [3]. The recent article published by Rudd et al. [4] is the first comprehensive global report on the epidemiology of sepsis. It assessed the burden of sepsis across 195 countries and territories within the framework of all 282 underlying causes of death, both sexes, and 23 age groups for the years 1990 to 2017 in the Global Burden of Diseases, Injuries, and Risk Factors Study (GBD) 2017 study. It is estimated that in 2017, there were 48.9 million cases and 11 million sepsis-related deaths worldwide, i.e., almost 20% of all global deaths. Approximately 85% of sepsis cases and sepsis-related deaths worldwide occurred in countries with low to middle sociodemographic indices that had much higher rates than those with higher indices. Nearly half of all sepsis-related deaths occur secondary to sepsis complicating an underlying injury or non-communicable disease. In 2017, almost half of all global sepsis cases occurred among children, with an estimated 20 million cases and 2.9 million global deaths in children under five years of age. The hospital mortality rate of sepsis was estimated to be 27% and mortality in ICU-treated sepsis was 42%. Among adult sepsis survivors, one in three died within a year, and one in six experienced significant, long-term morbidity [5]. Patients who survive sepsis often have long-term physical, psychological, and cognitive disabilities with significant health care and social implications.

Fleischmann-Struzek et al. [6] published an extensive systemic review analyzing the global burden of pediatric and neonatal sepsis. The review was based on 1270 studies published from 1979 to 2016. They performed the largest meta-analysis of population-based sepsis incidence in neonates and children, including 15 studies from 12 middle- and high-income countries on four continents. They estimated that 48 children per 100,000 population develop sepsis, 22 children per 100,000 population develop severe sepsis. Mortality ranged from 1.3% to 5.4% for sepsis, and 9–20% for severe sepsis. The population-level estimated for neonatal sepsis was 2202 per 100,000 live births, with mortality between 11% and 19%. This would translate to an incidence of 3 million cases of neonatal sepsis and 1.2 million cases of pediatric sepsis annually. These estimates are exploratory because of the considerable heterogeneity between data and the lack of population-based data from low-income and middle-income settings. Analyzing these alarming data, it is clear why the WHO, in 2017, listed sepsis as a key healthcare priority for the coming decade.

Sepsis is treatable, but early diagnosis is highly needed, due to significant clinical heterogeneity and the non-specificity of clinical symptoms. If it is not identified early and timely managed, sepsis may lead to severe and life-threatening complications such as septic shock, multiple organ failure, and death [7]. Early diagnosis is also important from an economic view since the earlier diagnosis of sepsis lowers the costs [8]. Sepsis-3 Task Force reiterates the concept that sepsis shall be identified using clinical criteria for life-threatening organ dysfunction and blood culture. Although blood culture has been considered the gold standard reference method for detecting and isolating pathogenic organisms from sterile body fluid specimens, its accuracy remains limited because of overall low diagnostic sensitivity, with high false negative rates in patients after initiation of antibiotic therapy, and in patients with severe localized infections or in the noninfectious cause of sepsis and preanalytical variables (inaccurate skin antisepsis, failure to use sterile gloves collection through central venous caterers, use of open blood collection systems, inadequate filling of blood culture bottles, long-term storage under inappropriate conditions, etc.). The drawbacks of blood culture are long turnaround time (its results are rarely available in a useful timeframe for decision-making), large sample volume, and frequent need for repeated testing [9, 10].

We have witnessed over the last years that an extensive variety of technologies for the identification of pathogens have been examined [11, 12]. Although some molecular diagnostic techniques, such as DNA/RNA rapid amplification followed by mass spectrometry or nuclear magnetic resonance are available and enable molecular identification of the causative organism in a few hours, limitations in their diagnostic performance still exist and must be overcome. Additional well-known drawbacks include: the need of dedicated often expensive equipment, high sensitivity of technique used for lysis and nucleic acids extraction, vulnerability to environmental contaminations, possible generation of false positive results due to deep-seated infections, doubts about the optimal sample matrix, interference from host nucleic acid and additional substances, amplification bias, off-target interactions, as well as to current limitedness and insufficient standardization of test panels [9].

Delays in the initiation of antimicrobial treatment are associated with a worse prognosis [13]. The current treatment guidelines for treating sepsis promulgate initiation of effective antibiotics within 1–3 h [14]. A large number of patients with sepsis still remain microbiologically undiagnosed in that period, thus, amplifying the risk of indiscriminate use of empiric antibiotics as broad-spectrum treatment. It contributes to the spread of antibiotic resistance genes, further exacerbating the emergence of multidrug-resistant microbial pathogens and secondary fungal infections [15]. Sometimes, empiric antibiotics are often administered to patients before arriving in the hospital and before exhibiting progressive signs of sepsis, thereby precluding an accurate microbial diagnosis by standard culture.

Due to explained limitations, there has been intense interest in identifying biomarkers of sepsis. Numerous serum/plasma sepsis biomarkers have been commercialized over the past decades. We are the witnesses that a growing body of literature over the last years revealed more than 250 sepsis biomarkers that offer utility for diagnosis, prognosis, early disease recognition, risk stratification, and appropriate treatment for patients with sepsis or suspected sepsis [16]. It is very well known that the ideal sepsis biomarker should be present at symptoms onset (or even earlier) and allow for an early diagnosis, should offer both high specificity and sensitivity for infections, be capable to identify the causative microorganism, be informative on the clinical course, provide valuable information on the prognosis, and guide therapeutic decisions. Additionally, the ideal biomarker should be non/invasive, easily measured by a single, widely available test, reproducible, accurate, with defined optimal cut-off(s), known release kinetics, and cost-effective [17]. Despite a large number of biomarkers studied, no single biomarker emerged as a consistently reliable indicator for diagnosis and prognosis of sepsis. Given that none of these biomarkers fulfill all features of ideal sepsis biomarker, it is not surprising that the Sepsis-3 definition consensus states the role of biomarkers in sepsis diagnosis remains undefined [1], Surviving Sepsis Campaign guidelines for the management of sepsis mention that sepsis biomarkers can complement clinical evaluation [18].

Recent evidence suggests that an increased concentration of some sepsis biomarkers more reliably reflects the systemic host response to infection. Only a few biomarkers were reported to have a role specifically related to sepsis pathophysiology, rather than to a more general inflammatory reaction. However, only a handful of these has reached the point of clinical availability, i.e., validation in clinical practice. The measurement of some sepsis biomarkers in addition to blood culture or molecular biology further improves the diagnostic management of patients with possible sepsis. It appears that some sepsis biomarkers are favorable markers for the evaluation of sepsis severity, for garnering valuable prognostic information, and guiding therapeutic decision-making i.e., antibiotic stewardship.

Among the emerging biomarkers of sepsis, the soluble CD14 subtype (sCD14-ST) also known as presepsin received increasing attention as one of the most promising. This chapter will summarize our current knowledge of presepsin with emphasis on its clinical usefulness as a diagnostic and prognostic biomarker in sepsis.

2. Soluble CD14 subtype (sCD14-ST)–presepsin

Presepsin, which is also known as soluble CD14 subtype (sCD14-ST) (64 amino-acids, 13 kDa) is a glycoprotein fragment mostly synthesized and released in general circulation by macrophages or monocytes/macrophages in response to infections [19, 20]. The CD14 receptor is a pattern recognition receptor in the innate immune response that has the ability to identify different pathogen-associated molecular pattern molecules of both Gram-positive and Gram-negative bacteria such as lipopolysaccharide, peptidoglycan, lipoteichoic acid, etc. The best-studied ligand is lipopolysaccharide (LPS) of Gram-negative bacteria [21, 22].

CD14 has two forms: membrane-bound CD14 (mCD14) and soluble CD14 (sCD14). The first, mCD14 receptor (356 amino acids, 55-kDa), is a membrane glycoprotein [23], whose C-terminal leader sequence of 28–30 amino acids is replaced by a glycosyl phosphatidylinositol (GPI) anchor after translation [24]. Thus, mCD14 is anchored to the cellular membrane through GPI linkage. It does not possess an intracellular tail; it is not a transmembrane protein and is unable to transmit a signal by itself. Although CD14 is detected predominantly on the surface of myeloid-lineage cells; however, low amounts are also found in non-myeloid cells, e.g., hepatocytes, adipocytes, corneal, and intestinal epithelial cells. The circulating soluble form-sCD14 is found in plasma and is produced by mCD14 fall-off or cell secretion [25].

Various stimuli induce shedding of the GPI anchored mCD14, probably mediated by serine proteases such as leucocyte elastase [26] resulting in sCD14 with a molecular mass of 48–49 kDa. Some CD14 molecules stored intracellularly escape GPI anchor attachment and keep the C-terminal leader sequence, resulting in sCD14 with a molecular weight of 55–56 kDa [27]. After that, sCD14 is cleaved by cathepsin D and other proteases in plasma or the phagolysosome and the truncated 13-kDa form of sCD14, called presepsin is generated and released into circulation.

After being released into circulation, lipopolysaccharide (LPS, endotoxin) of Gram-negative bacteria (the prevailing cause of severe sepsis in humans) binds to a specific plasma protein known as lipopolysaccharide-binding protein (LBP). LBP presents LPS to CD14 which is recruited to the receptor after ligand binding. The LPS/LBP complex after binding to CD14, mediated by myeloid differentiation factor 2 (MD2), finally binds to Toll-like receptor 4 (TLR4), resulting in its activation. Both membrane-bound and soluble CD14 can transfer the LPS molecule to the TLR4/MD-2 complex. TLR4 activation sequentially triggers two signaling cascades. The first one is the MyD88-signaling pathway at the plasma membrane, and the second is the TRIF-dependent signaling pathway. Dimerization of the receptor complex induces the assembly of TIRAP, MyD88, and IRAK kinases in a submembrane signaling complex called the myddosome at the TIR domain of TLR4 inducing a signaling pathway inducing expression of genes encoding pro-inflammatory cytokines (IL-6, TNF-α, etc.). The MyD88-dependent signaling is followed by internalization of TLR4 in endosomes. Simultaneously, TIRAP and MyD88 dissociate from the membrane allowing TLR4 to bind in the endosome the second set of TIR-containing adaptor proteins, TRAM and TRIF, controlling the production of type I interferons, CCL5/RANTES. Via activated NF-κB TLR4 also contributes to the activation of the cytosolic NLRP3 inflammasome [28]. Notably, while CD14 is marginally important for MyD88-dependent TNFα expression, it is essential for TRIF-mediated IFN expression because it regulates TLR4 endocytosis [29].

2.1 Kinetic of presepsin release

The kinetics of presepsin is extraordinarily rapid in blood. Presepsin levels increase in the blood within 2 h after the onset of any infection, with a maximum concentration after 3 h, and tended to decrease on day 7. The half-life of presepsin is 4–5 h at the plasma level [30]. In 2008, Nakamura et al. [31] in an experimental peritonitis model of sepsis in rabbits using cecum ligation and puncture, detected presepsin in the blood of animals 2 h after initiation of the procedure. Presepsin levels peaked at 3 h and decreased 4–8 h after initiation of the procedure. In 2016, Chenevier-Gobeaux et al. [32] measured presepsin levels after LPS stimulation in peripheral mononuclear cells (PMNC) and human cell line of mononuclear cells (THP-1), and found that In THP1 cells, presepsin levels increase after 1 h, reaching a peak after 3 h, and decreasing at 4 h after LPS exposure. In PMNC, exposure to LPS induced an increase of median presepsin levels as early as hour 1, concomitantly to IL-6 synthesis.

3. Measurement of soluble CD14 subtype (sCD14-ST)–presepsin

Different methods have been developed for the determination of presepsin. The first, presepsin concentrations were measured using a two-step sandwich enzyme-linked immunosorbent assay (ELISA). Large recombinant CD14 antigen (S286C, approximately 40 kDa) was used as standard. The dynamic range of the two-step assay was 3–150 ng/ml. The total assay time was 4 h. This test was sufficient to evaluate presepsin as a diagnostic marker for sepsis, but it lacked the speed and accuracy that are required for routine presepsin tests in ICU. Soon after, Shirakawa et al. [33] modified a traditional two-step into one-step ELISA. The standard used in the one-step method was recombinant presepsin, the sample dilution step was eliminated and two new anti-presepsin antibodies were used: F1106-13-3 monoclonal antibody as the capture antibody and S68 polyclonal antibody as the detection antibody. The dynamic range of the one-step assay was 0.05–3.00 ng/ml. The total assay time was 1.5 h. This assay is suitable for clinical practice [33]. However, this method has low linearity and several endogenous (rheumatoid factor, cross-reactive substances, complement) and exogenous (specimen hemolysis, bacteria, and iatrogenic tube contamination) interfering factors [34].

In 2011, Okamura and Yokoi [35] have developed and evaluated the analytical and clinical performance of the highly sensitive, fully automated PATHFAST Presepsin test. This test performed on the PATHFAST instrument (Pathfast, Mitsubishi Chemical Medicine Corporation, Tokyo, Japan) is based on a noncompetitive chemiluminescent enzyme immunoassay combined with Magtration® technology. The principle of the test is as follows. The patient sample is dispensed into the reagent cartridge. The instrument combines the patient sample, the anti-presepsin monoclonal antibody-coated magnetic particles, and the alkaline phosphatase-labeled anti-presepsin polyclonal antibody and incubates the mixture for 5 min at 37°C. During this incubation, the analyte in the patient sample binds to the antibody on the coated particles, and the alkaline phosphatase conjugate binds to the analyte-antibody coated-particle. After the incubation, the instrument performs Bound/Free (B/F) separation using Magtration® technology to remove any excess unbound reagents, chemiluminescent substrate (CDP-Star Chemiluminescent Substrate) was added. The substrate is catalyzed by the bound alkaline phosphatase, which results in the emission of photons. The photo-multiplier tube in the PATHFAST instrument detects the photons that are emitted during the reaction. The chemiluminescent count is converted to analyte concentration values by the instrument based on the master calibration curve for the reagent lot [36]. According to the manufacturer's data assay range is 20–20,000 pg/ml. The assay reveals its result within 15 min in six samples simultaneously, using a sample volume of 100 μl. The calibrator for the PATHFAST Presepsin assay is recombinant presepsin (13 kDa). The sensitivity of the PATHFAST Presepsin assay was sufficient to detect the presepsin concentrations of the healthy group. It was higher than the recently reported one-step ELISA [37]. The PATHFAST Presepsin assay correlated well with a previously reported two-step presepsin ELISA [33]. PATHFAST is applicable for use in the Emergency Department (ED), ICU, and surgical wards. No interference of presepsin was noticed for bilirubin, hemoglobin, lipids, triglyceride, or rheumatoid factors [35].

Recently, evaluation results of a new automated one-step sandwich chemiluminescent enzyme immunoassay for presepsin measurement on Sysmex HISCL-5000 (Sysmex, Japan) was published [38]. Briefly, biotinylated anti-presepsin monoclonal antibodies specifically react with presepsin in the sample. This complex binds to streptavidin-coated magnetic particles (MPs). After bound/free separation, alkaline phosphatase (ALP)-labeled anti-presepsin monoclonal antibodies specifically bind to the presepsin on an MP. Then, the ALP on the MP breaks down the CDP-Star® chemiluminescent substrate which produces a luminescent signal. Assay samples were tested undiluted, with an analytical measurement range of–30,000 pg/ml. Turn-around-time for measuring the first sample was 17 min and the total processing capacity was around 200 tests per hour. For the first time, Sysmex HISCL-5000 and PATHFAST presepsin tests were performed, and a high significant correlation was found. Also, SCD14-ST concentration picogram/milliliter (pg/ml) can be measured using CL1200i (Mindray, Shenzen, China), according to manufacturer protocol based on sandwich chemiluminescent enzyme immunoassay. The measurement range of the assay was 20–20,000 pg/ml [39].

4. Presepsin values in the reference population

Few studies measured presepsin concentrations in the reference population. They found that presepsin is present in low concentrations in healthy individuals. Mean concentrations were in range between 21.8 and 312 pg/ml, median was around 200 pg/ml [35, 37, 40–47].

However, current literature suggests an operational cut-off for the decision making process at the 95th percentile value. However, this value can be measured with enough statistical confidence (>95% CI) only if the studied population is >300 volunteers. Thus, this detection remains to be established for presepsin use today. Okamura and Yokoi [35] determined presepsin in the heparinized plasma of 127 healthy volunteers. The 95th percentile value was for plasma/whole blood 333 pg/ml/314 pg/ml. Carpio et al. [48] measured presepsin concentrations in EDTA plasma samples of 123 healthy volunteers and revealed a PSEP range of 58–339 ng/l and a 95% reference interval with an upper and lower reference limit of 236 ng/l (90% CI 222–250 ng/l) and 24 ng/l (90% CI 10–38 ng/l), respectively. Males showed slightly higher values than females. Median values were 133 and 101 ng/l, respectively ($P = 0.0435$).

Few studies published presepsin cut-off levels (pg/ml) expressed as medians (minimum-maximum) in healthy control infants, preterm and term infants. Mussap et al. [49] enrolled 26 consecutive non-septic preterm newborns with gestational age (GA) between 26 and 36 weeks admitted to NICU after the first day of life for various severe diseases. The obtained median presepsin value was 578 ng/l, the authors finally indicate preliminary reference ranges for preterm newborns 255–1144 ng/l. They did not find a correlation between GA and sCD14-ST presepsin blood levels between 26 and 36 weeks and they suggested adopting a unique reference range for preterm newborns. Pugni et al. [50] recently performed the first study that determined presepisn reference ranges in a large group (684 neonates) of term and preterm neonates (484 born at term and 200 were preterm (24–36 weeks' gestation). In term infants, presepsin median value was 603.5 pg/ml (interquartile range: 466.5–791 pg/ml; 5th and 95th centiles: 315 and 1178 pg/ml, respectively). In preterm infants, presepsin median value was slightly higher, equal to 620 pg/ml (interquartile range: 503–864 pg/ml; 5th and 95th centiles: 352 and 1370 pg/ml, respectively). The determined reference ranges of presepsin were much higher than those seen in healthy adults. No correlation between presepsin levels and postnatal age was observed, as well as no significant difference was demonstrated in preterm neonates at different gestational ages. None of the variables analyzed affected presepsin levels to a clinically significant extent. Poggi et al. [51] analyzed presepsin values in 183 preterm infants with ≤32 weeks of GA during the first 48 h of life and measured presepsin at four different time points. Presepsin median value within 6, 12, 24, and 48 h of birth was 583, 614, 604 and 513 ng/l, respectively. Presepsin values were negatively associated with GA at the first three time points. Recently, Nur Ergor et al. [52] in 144 neonates born at 24–42 weeks' gestation revealed, for the first time, the reference ranges of presepsin in healthy term and preterm neonates without infection with respect to gestational and postnatal age, sex, and body weight. Presepsin measurements included cord blood levels and serum levels on postnatal days 1, 3, 5, 7, 14, 21, and 28. The presepsin values corresponding to the 10th percentile ranged from 240.8 pg/ml (on day 1) to 129.9 pg/ml (on day 28), whereas those corresponding to the 90th percentile ranged from 725.8 pg/ml (on day 1) to 471.6 pg/ml (on day 28). Significantly higher presepsin levels were observed in cesarean deliveries than in spontaneous deliveries (P: 0.012 to <0.001), in gestational ages ≤32 weeks than in gestational ages ≥37 weeks (P: <0.05 to <0.001), and in cases with a maternal history of chorioamnionitis than in those without (*P*: <0.05 to <0.001).

In the pediatric setting, mean presepsin plasma levels in healthy infants are much higher (720 ng/l) than in healthy adults, probably due to the passage after birth from the intrauterine environment to the new external environment rich in foreign antigens, which activates the innate immune system [53].

5. Presepsin values interpretation

Presepsin values are usually interpreted as follows [20]:

Presepsin, pg/ml	Diagnosis
<200	Sepsis excluded
<300	Systemic infection improbable
<500	Sepsis probable
<1000	Significant risk of severe sepsis
≥1000	High risk of severe sepsis/septic shock equivalent to SOFA≥8

Special care must be taken in interpreting altered presepsin levels. Presepsin concentrations increase with age, and the interpretation of presepsin is altered in elderly patients. Special attention should be paid on newborn presepsin values. Presepsin is a small protein, filtered by the glomerulus and reabsorbed and completely catabolized within proximal tubular cells. Since the kidney is involved in the presepsin excretion, the presepsin plasma levels are increased in patients with renal failure. Presepsin levels could rise above the cut-off value in patients with renal dysfunction, and in this case, presepsin concentrations should be interpreted with caution. For this reason, the cut-offs must be adapted in patients with chronic kidney disease and/or on hemodialysis treatment [43, 54].

Presepsin is also influenced by translocation of the intestinal microbial flora [55]. As presepsin is not only excreted through the kidney but also in the hepatobiliary system, its abnormalities may therefore be related to higher levels of presepsin level. Cholestasis significantly increases biliary enzymes, suggesting that presepsin is elevated in patients with cholestasis. Lin et al. [56] indicated an association between presepsin and the severity of cholangitis. This may indicate that an increase in the total bilirubin is associated with the presepsin level. A markedly high presepsin level may be associated with obstructive jaundice [57]. These findings highlight the need of establishing adapted cut-offs for specific populations/conditions.

6. Presepsin as a diagnostic and prognostic marker

Since 2005, when it was first reported that presepsin was increased in patients with sepsis [37], suggesting its utility as an early diagnostic marker of sepsis, numerous studies have been performed with the aim to evaluate the usefulness of presepsin as a diagnostic and prognostic biomarker in sepsis. Also, few meta-analyses have been published evaluating the diagnostic and prognostic value of presepsin. The first meta-analysis published in 2015 mainly focused on validating the diagnostic value of presepsin in adult sepsis, and the newer analyses examined the prognostic values of presepsin value for adult sepsis. Recently published meta-analyses were performed mainly on neonates, examining the diagnostic and prognostic value of presepsin in sepsis. Some of them analyzed the prognostic value of presepsin in comparison and combination with traditional sepsis biomarkers such as C-reactive protein (CRP) and procalcitonin (PCT).

6.1 Presepsin as a diagnostic marker

Numerous studies, mainly conducted in the last decade, have assessed the diagnostic value of presepsin for sepsis, with conflicting results. The studies reported that presepsin efficiency depends on the cut-off used. Different cut-off values reported by these studies may be caused by the heterogeneity of the studies in the clinical setting (ED vs. ICU), the sepsis criteria adopted (before or after Sepsis-3), study design (prospective vs. retrospective), comorbidities, or the type of sample used (plasma vs. whole blood vs. serum) for measurement of presepsin. Optimal cut-off values (sensitivity and specificity, respectively) to discriminate sepsis from non-sepsis were 907 (70%, 83%) [30], 686 (47%, 91%) [58], 729 (81%, 63%) [59], 600 (79%, 62%) [60], 542 (77%, 76%) [61], 430 (88%, 82%) [45], 466 (90%, 55%) pg/ml [62]. In the study by Shozushima et al. [40] the optimal cut-off value of presepsin was 399 pg/ml, until, in Liu et al. [42], the optimal cut-off value of presepsin was 317 pg/ml.

Several studies revealed the potential greater utility of presepsin over PCT in the early diagnosis of sepsis. Some studies have shown that presepsin has diagnostic and prognostic power substantially similar to PCT, but, unlike PCT, presepsin increases earlier in bacterial infection and can be measured effectively and accurately within 15 min using a POCT analyzer. Rare studies showed the opposite results.

In a 2013 prospective cohort study [42] in consecutive ED patients with at least two diagnostic criteria for SIRS in the ED (prior Sepsis-3), presepsin was the superior diagnostic marker of sepsis than PCT. In patients with bacterial and non-bacterial infection in acute abdominal conditions, Vodnik et al. [63] reported that presepsin discriminates SIRS from sepsis much better than PCT, CRP, or WBC. They also reported that presepsin was superior to PCT and CRP in discriminating sepsis from SIRS in acute abdominal conditions. Kweon et al. [45] found higher diagnostic accuracy of presepsin compared to PCT, IL6, and CRP in patients presenting to the ED with suspected sepsis. Hou et al. [64] reported that presepsin had a higher diagnostic value compared with both PCT and CRP patients with nephrolithiasis presenting with SIRS. In another 2015 study, using a cut-off of 413 ng/L for diagnosing bacterial infections in ICU patients, Godnic et al. [65] reported that presepsin has a higher area under the curve (AUC) compared to PCT (0.705 vs. 0.630) but lower than CRP (0.705 vs. 0.734). In a study conducted on ICU patients, presepsin was effective in predicting sepsis with sensitivity and specificity values of 84.6% and 62.5%, respectively, which were significantly related to the APACHE II score (P-value = 0.016).

The multicenter prospective study that included 207 suspected sepsis patients demonstrated that presepsin is useful for the diagnosis of bacterial infections as PCT [46]. The cutoff value of presepsin for discrimination of bacterial and nonbacterial infectious diseases was determined to be 600 pg/ml, with sensitivity 87.8% and specificity 81.4%. A study performed by de Guadiana Romualdo et al. [59] in 2014, has included 226 patients admitted to the ED with SIRS criteria, of which 37 had positive blood culture (bacteremic SIRS group) and 189 had negative blood culture (non-bacteremic SIRS group). They showed that presepsin values can be used to rule out the diagnosis of bacteremia in SIRS patients in the ED setting (cut-off value 729 pg/ml, sensitivity 81.1%, specificity 63%, PPV 30%, and NVP 94.4%). In this study, presepsin showed a similar diagnostic accuracy to PCT. A few years later, the same authors examined 223 patients admitted in ED with suspected sepsis, using two cut-offs (312 and 849 ng/l) and found sensitivity 97.1% and 67.1% and specificity 16.9% and 80.8%, respectively. They also reported that the diagnostic accuracy of presepsin does not improve that of PCT [58]. Cakır Madenci et al. [61] revealed that presepsin levels had comparable performances with PCT, CRP, and WBC levels in burn sepsis. In 2016, Alli et al. [30] and Leli et al. [66] in prospective cohort studies of patients with SIRS/suspected sepsis/healthy controls, and patients with suspected sepsis, respectively showed that presepsin and PCT had good diagnostic accuracy, whereas presepsin was superior to CRP.

Contenti et al. [67] using Sepsis-3 reported that presepsin can effectively discriminate sepsis from non-infectious SIRS and that presepsin and PCT were superior to CRP and lactate in discriminating sepsis, including shock, from non-sepsis with SIRS and a SOFA score ≥ 2. The study showed that the AUC values used to discriminate sepsis from non-sepsis were 0.88 for presepsin. The sensitivity, specificity, positive predictive value, negative predictive value, and accuracy of presepsin for diagnosing sepsis (including shock) using a cut-off value of 508 pg/ml were 87%, 86%, 93%, 76%, and 87%, respectively. A recently published study by Lee et al. [68] performed the largest prospective observational study on the diagnostic value of presepsin in non-infectious organ failure, sepsis, and septic shock, in accordance with the latest Sepsis-3 definitions. They reported that presepsin has good accuracy in discriminating sepsis from non-infectious organ failure and had fair accuracy in discriminating septic shock from sepsis. Presepsin best cut-off to discriminate sepsis and non-infectious organ failure was 582 pg/ml (sensitivity 70.1%, specificity 89.4%, AUC 0.877, $P < 0.001$) and sepsis and septic shock 1285 pg/ml (sensitivity 50.4%, specificity 76.6%, AUC 0.618, $P < 0.001$). The discriminating power of presepsin was comparable with that of PCT among patients with non-infectious organ failure/sepsis/septic shock.

Two center studies published in 2013 [60], including patients in the ED with suspected sepsis/septic shock, and patients with SIRS without clinical evidence of infection, found that the diagnostic accuracy of presepsin was generally lower than PCT. Sargentini et al. [69] showed that presepsin can accurately differentiate septic and non/septic patients in ICU, but it is inferior compared to PCT. At the same time, Claessens et al. [41] also confirmed that presepsin was less accurate than PCT to predict bacteraemia in patients with acute pyelonephritis and bacteremia.

The level of presepsin will rise significantly in early-onset sepsis. Whether presepsin can indicate Gram-positive and Gram-negative bacterial infection is still controversial. Lu et al. [70] reported that the cut-off value of presepsin for discrimination of sepsis and nonbacterial infectious SIRS was determined to be 407 pg/ml, with a sensitivity 98.6% and specificity 82.6% in patients with sepsis and SIRS in the ED. They compared presepsin levels in septic patients infected with various kinds of pathogens and did not find a significant difference in patients with Gram-positive, Gram-negative, mixed (bacterial and fungal), fungal infection and unknown infection. But, presepsin was significantly different between Gram-positive and Gram-negative bacterial infections ($P < 0.05$), enabling distinguishing Gram-positive and Gram-negative bacterial infections. Besides, Masson et al. [71] in 997 patients with severe sepsis or septic shock in the multicenter Albumin Italian Outcome Sepsis

(ALBIOS) trial reported that patients infected with Gram-negative bacterial infections had higher levels of presepsin than those with Gram-positive infections. Also, presepsin concentration was significantly higher in patients with bacterial infection (according to the site or blood culture) than in those with negative culture or in those with no culture available. However, Endo et al. [46] have gained the opposite results; there was no significant difference between Gram-positive and Gram-negative bacterial infections, as well as no significant differences in presepsin levels between the blood culture-positive and culture-negative groups.

It was found that presepsin should also be useful for the diagnosis of bacteremia in hematological patients undergoing stem cell transplants with a cutoff value of 218 pg/ml [72]. The same authors two years later in another study of hematological patients undergoing chemotherapy reported that presepsin is useful for the differentiation between bacterial and fungal infection. They found that elevated CRP in conjunction with presepsin within the normal reference range was in favor of fungal infection in this group of immunocompromized individuals [73].

Klouche et al. [62] reported greater specificity of presepsin and PCT in combination for the diagnosis of sepsis, septic shock and pneumonia, compared to using PCT alone or presepsin alone. In 2016, Plesko et al. [74] reported that in hematologic patients the association of presepsin with IL-6 increases sensitivity compared to the use of presepsin alone in detecting sepsis, while the association of presepsin with PCT and CRP did not show better accuracy than presepsin alone in detecting sepsis in this type of patients. Chan et al. [75] reported that a cut-off value of 1025 pg/ml presepsin had 83% specificity and 85% sensitivity for the diagnosis of sepsis. This case–control study (60 patients admitted to ICU with sepsis/60 controls) showed that presepsin and sTREM-1 were more sensitive for the diagnosis of sepsis compared to PCT and CRP. The most accurate indicator was a composite biomarker of presepsin and sTREM-1. In 2015, Carpio et al. [48] performed a single-center prospective observational study (120 patients with SIRS or sepsis criteria (before Sepsis-3) and 123 healthy controls) confirmed that presepsin at a cut-off of 581 ng/l is effective in diagnosing sepsis, graduating severity of disease and differentiating between SIRS and sepsis in ED, with the sensitivity of 61% and specificity of 100%. The performance of presepsin varies according to the cut-off considered: using a cut-off of 273 ng/l, a sensitivity of 95.5% and specificity of 21.7% were found, while using a cut-off of 686 ng/l, these values were 46.5% and 91.3%, respectively. This study showed that the combination of presepsin and MEDS score improved discriminatory power compared with presepsin or MEDS score alone. In a single center study of 250 patients older than 75 years admitted in ED with suspected sepsis, Ruangsomboon et al. [76] revealed that presepsin had a similar diagnostic accuracy as PCT and the early warning score. Presepsin was found to be an accurate biomarker for sepsis diagnosis in geriatric persons older than 75 years in combination with PCT and the early warning score.

Among the biomarkers identified as a potential diagnostic markers for neonatal sepsis, presepsin seems to be promising. A recently published review analyzed literature data about presepsin as a biomarker for the diagnosis of neonatal sepsis [77]. In 2015, 13 studies [78–90] were assessed presepsin accuracy as an early diagnostic biomarker of sepsis in infants preterm and term infants. Ten out of the 13, performed longitudinal presepsin monitoring from birth up to the first week of life. Cut-offs were 300–987 ng/l sensitivity 67–100%, specificity 75–100%, Presepsin accuracy as a diagnostic test for perinatal sepsis, and a comparison with the standard of care parameters such as CRP and PCT was provided. The research strategy allowed for the selection of seven studies in which presepsin, CRP, and PCT accuracy were investigated according to different outcomes [78, 81, 82, 84, 86–88]. It was shown that presepsin is a valuable diagnostic test for sepsis (EOS and LOS) with higher sensitivity and specificity values than PCT and CRP [81, 87, 88], or similarly accurate as a diagnostic test of EOS to CRP and PCT [78, 86].

6.1.1 Systematic reviews and meta-analyses

The first comprehensive meta-analysis [91], published in 2015 included 11 studies [37, 40, 42, 45, 46, 55, 59–61, 63, 92] (1630 sepsis cases, 1422 controls) with heterogenous inclusion criteria. It revealed the overall diagnostic sensitivity of presepsin for sepsis was 0.83 (95% CI: 0.77–0.88) and the specificity was 0.78 (95% CI: 0.72–0.83). The diagnostic odds ratio was 18 (95% CI: 11–30). The area under the summary receiver operating characteristic curve (sROC) was 0.88 (95% CI: 0.84–0.90), until the positive and negative likelihood ratios of presepsin for revealing sepsis were 3.9 (95% CI: 2.9–5.0) and 0.21 (95% CI: 0.15–0.30), respectively. When presepsin was introduced as a diagnostic test for sepsis, sepsis probability increased from 56% (pre-test probability among all subjects) to 81% (post-test probability for a positive result). Presepsin is an effective adjunct biomarker for sepsis diagnosis, but presepsin alone is insufficient to rule out or confirm sepsis, and its results should be interpreted within the clinical context.

In 2015, Wu et al. [93] published a systematic review and meta-analysis of 10 trials (9 studies) [40, 42, 44, 45, 55, 60, 63, 94, 95], conducted in internal care unit, critical care unit, in the emergency department in Eastern Asia and Western Europe. It included 1320 sepsis patients, 512 with SIRS of non-infectious origin, and 327 healthy persons. The pooled sensitivity of presepsin for sepsis was 0.78 (0.76–0.80), pooled specificity was 0.83 (0.80–0.85), pooled diagnostic odds ratio was 21.73 (12.81–36.86), pooled positive likelihood ratio was 4.63 (3.27–6.55), and pooled negative likelihood ratio was 0.22 (0.16–0.30). Wu et al. [93] found similar sensitivity (0.85 vs. 0.84), but lower specificity in the cut-off values greater than 700 pg/ml studies, compared to values smaller than 700 pg/ml studies (0.59 vs. 0.80). This meta-analysis showed that presepsin could be helpful in sepsis early diagnosis, and has only moderate diagnostic value in differentiating sepsis from other non-septic inflammatory conditions.

In the same year, meta-analysis [96] of eight studies [42, 44–46, 59, 60, 63, 97] from Europe and Asia were published. It included 1815 patients, from whom SIRS criteria were fulfilled in 1690 patients (1165 patients with sepsis and 525 patients with non-infectious SIRS)). This meta-analysis revealed very good diagnostic accuracy of presepsin (AUC 0.89 (95% CI: 0.86–0.92)) for the diagnosis of sepsis in SIRS patients. The pooled sensitivity was 0.86 (95% CI: 0.79–0.91), specificity was 0.78 (95% CI: 0.68–0.85), diagnostic odds ratio 22 (95% CI: 10–48), positive likelihood ratio 3.8 (95% CI: 2.6–5.7), and negative likelihood ratio 0.18 (95% CI: 0.11–0.28). According to this meta-analysis, presepsin cannot be recommended as the single definitive test for diagnosis of sepsis.

The systematic review and meta-analysis of Zheng et al. [98] included eight studies [42, 44–46, 59, 60, 65, 97] with 1757 patients who evaluated the accuracy of presepsin for the diagnosis of sepsis from SIRS patients. The pooled sensitivity was 0.77 (95% CI 0.75–0.80), specificity 0.73 (95% CI 0.69–0.77), and diagnostic odds ratio was 14.25 (95% CI 8.66–23.42). The summary receiver operating characteristic curve (sROC) AUC was 0.8598, indicating that the presepsin had a moderate diagnostic efficiency.

A bivariate meta-analysis of Tong et al. [99] of 11 publications [40, 42, 44–46, 60, 61, 63, 92, 97, 100] examined the use of presepsin to diagnose sepsis with 3106 subjects. The sensitivity was 0.83 (95% CI 0.77–0.88), specificity 0.81 (95% CI 0.74–0.87), DDR 21.56 (95% CI 10.59–43.88), PLR 4.43 (95% CI 3.05–6.43), NLR 0.21 (95% CI 0.14–0.30). The area under the curve was 0.89 (95% CI 0.86–0.92). Estimated positive and negative post-probability values for a sepsis prevalence of 20% were 53% and 5%, respectively. This analysis showed the valuable role of presepsin in the diagnosis of sepsis, but stated that presepsin values should be interpreted carefully in a clinical context considering traditional markers.

Li et al. [101] conducted a large systematic review and meta-analysis of nine studies [40, 46, 48, 59, 60, 63, 65, 97, 100] comprised of 1510 participants to evaluate the diagnostic value of potential biomarkers (among them presepsin) for the differential diagnosis of non-infectious SIRS and sepsis. The obtained sensitivity for presepsin was 0.84 (95% CI 0.79–0.88), specificity (0.77 (95% CI 0.68–0.84), AUC was 0.88 (95% CI 0.85–0.90). It was shown that presepsin has moderate diagnostic utility in differentiating sepsis from SIRS. This analysis showed a similar diagnostic accuracy of presepsin in detecting sepsis as PCT, CRP, IL6, sTREM-1, LBP, and CD64.

Next year Wu et al. [102] published a systematic review and meta-analysis of 18 studies [40, 42, 44–46, 48, 55, 58–63, 65, 92, 97, 100, 103] including 3470 patients with the aim to assess the accuracy of presepsin for the diagnosis of sepsis in adult patients and compare the performance of presepsin, and traditionally examined biomarkers CRP, PCT. The pooled diagnosis sensitivity of presepsin for sepsis was 0.84 (95% CI 0.80–0.87), specificity was 0.76 (95% CI 0.67–0.82), the pooled DOR was 16 (95% CI 10–25), PLR 3.4 (95% CI 2.5–4.6), NLR 0.22 (95% CI 0.17–0.27), and AUC 0.88 (95% CI 0.85–0.90). It showed that presepsin is a good predictor for sepsis but there are no significant variations compared to PCT or CRP. Presepsin has similar diagnostic accuracy as PCT or CRP.

Although Hayashida et al. [104] in 2016, first decided to conduct a systematic review and meta-analysis to evaluate the diagnostic accuracy of PCT and presepsin to a reference standard of sepsis/infection and to compare the diagnostic accuracy with each other in critically ill adult patients, their work was published three years later [105]. It included 10 studies [30, 44, 46, 59, 61, 62, 65, 66, 106, 107] that enrolled 1389 patients with established infection in the critical care setting. It was focused only on studies evaluating participants with critical illnesses, such as acute respiratory distress syndrome and sepsis, but not healthy volunteers. Diagnostic accuracy in detecting infection is similar for PCT and presepsin (sensibility 0.80 and 0.84, specificity 0.75 and 0.73, respectively). It was shown that both biomarkers are useful for early diagnosis of sepsis and reduction of mortality in critically ill adults. It was shown that the diagnostic accuracy of both biomarkers in detecting infection was similar, also both are useful for early diagnosis of sepsis and reduction of mortality in critically ill adults.

Few meta-analyses regarding presepsin diagnostic accuracy in detecting neonatal sepsis were recently published. The first meta-analyses performed by Bellos et al. [108] evaluated the diagnostic accuracy of presepsin in neonates with suspected sepsis. This meta-analysis consisted of 11 studies [80, 84, 85, 87, 88, 90, 109–113] with a total number of 783 neonates (391 with neonatal sepsis, 392 controls). The pooled sensitivity of presepsin for the prediction of neonatal sepsis was 0.91 (95% CI [0.87–0.93]), pooled specificity was 0.91 (95% CI [0.88–0.94]), with a diagnostic odds ratio of 170.28 (95% CI [51.13–567.11]) and the AUC was 0.9751 (SE 0.0117). A head-to-head comparison with AUC values of CRP (0.9748 vs. 0.8580) and PCT (0.9596 vs. 0.7831) revealed that presepsin was more sensitive in detecting neonatal sepsis.

According to this meta-analysis, presepsin can help clinicians in identifying neonates at risk. Ruan et al. [114] performed a meta-analysis of 28 studies (2661participants) with the aim to compare the diagnostic accuracy of PCT, CRP, PCT combined with CRP (PCT + CRP), and presepsin in diagnosing neonatal sepsis. A total of six studies [84, 85, 87, 88, 90, 115] enrolling 463 neonates were included in this presepsin meta-analysis. The pooled sensitivity of presepsin (0.94 (95% CI 0.80–0.99)), the pooled NLR of presepsin (0.06 (95% CI 0.02–0.23)) and the AUC for presepsin (0.99 (95% CI 0.98–1.00)). The main finding of this meta-analysis was that presepsin alone or PCT plus CRP have better diagnostic power than CRP and PCT alone in neonatal sepsis. One of the largest reviews and meta-analyses [116] investigating the diagnostic accuracy of presepsin in detecting sepsis, performed on neonates include nine [78, 80, 83–85, 87, 90, 111, 113] high-quality studies, comprising 712 neonates. Meta-analysis results showed an overall sensitivity of 90% and an overall specificity of 90%, with an AUC of 0.968, indicating a high level of diagnostic accuracy in detecting neonatal sepsis. The pooled sensitivity was 0.90 (95% CI 0.86–0.93), pooled specificity was 0.90 (95% CI 0.86–0.93), the pooled DOR was 120.94 (95% CI 40.11–364.69), and AUC was 0.968 (SE 0.0136). Using cut-off values <600 ng/l, sensitivity was 0.93, specificity of 0.81 and AUC 0.8195, while using a threshold >600 ng/l, sensitivity was 0.87, specificity 0.97, with higher diagnostic accuracy (AUC 0.976). Diagnostic accuracy of presepsin resulted high in detection of neonatal sepsis. Even though it cannot be recommended as a single diagnostic test, presepsin could be a helpful and valuable biomarker in neonates with suspected sepsis.

However, these meta-analyses analyzed together studies that included EOS and LOS. They did not take into account that different timing of presepsin measurements may affect results and that a single cut-off value for EOS and LOS may be inappropriate, as presepsin values change during the first month of life [52]. Patient populations may also significantly differ, because LOS occurrence is definitely prevalent in hospitalized preterm newborns, and gestational age affects presepsin values [51].

Van Maldeghem et al. [117], in a published systematic review and meta-analysis, for the first time, evaluated the differences in diagnostic accuracy of presepsin between EOS and LOS. Twelve articles [49, 50, 80, 83–85, 87, 90, 109, 111, 113, 118] were included in the systematic review and ten in the meta-analysis. At sepsis onset, a consequently higher level of sCD14-ST was found in septic neonates compared to healthy controls with significantly higher levels in LOS compared to EOS. sCD14-ST levels increase in the first 24 h in EOS, but not in LOS. This underlines the importance to consider EOS and LOS as two different disease entities. Optimal cut-off values ranged from 305 to 672 ng/l for EOS cases vs. healthy controls. The pooled sensitivity was 81% (95% CI 0.76–0.85), pooled specificity 86% (95% CI 0.81–0.89) with an AUC of 0.9412 (SE 0.1178). In LOS optimal cut-off values ranged from 801 to 885 ng/l with a pooled sensitivity of 81% (95% CI 0.74–0.86) and a pooled specificity of 100% (95% CI 0.98–1.00). An AUC and sROC were not estimable in LOS because of the low number of studies.

Recently published the largest systematic review and meta-analysis on presepsin diagnostic performance in the neonatal population [119], and for the first time specifically assessed presepsin accuracy for the diagnosis of neonatal EOS. Twelve studies [79, 80, 83, 84, 109–111, 118, 120–123] and 828 newborns (including 460 with EOS and the rest uninfected) met the inclusion criteria for the primary analysis (positive blood culture). Ten of the studies included a mix of EOS and LOS, four only included infants born at term, two were restricted to preterm infants, and the rest had a mix. Half of the studies were performed in Egypt, while the remaining were conducted in

Europe and Asia. Presepsin had a pooled sensitivity of 0.93 for the primary analysis of culture-proven sepsis (95% CI 0.86–0.96), a pooled specificity of 0.91 (95% CI 0.85–0.95), and a pooled diagnostic odds ratio (DOR) of 131.7 (95% CI 54.9–310.9). Presepsin showed high pooled sensitivity and specificity; presepsin specificity was influenced by the inclusion of only early-onset or all neonatal sepsis. Accuracy was not affected by gestational age, test type, country of the study, or risk of bias of the included studies. The secondary analysis included 23 studies [78–80, 83, 84, 86–88, 109–113, 115, 118, 120–127] that met the broader criteria for sepsis (either positive blood culture or clinical sepsis) and involved 1866 newborns (1040 newborns with EOS and the rest uninfected), with seven of the trials involving only newborns with EOS produced similar results. Results of the secondary analysis were similar, with a pooled sensitivity of 0.93 (95% CI 0.89–0.96), a pooled specificity of 0.91 (95% CI 0.87–0.94), and a pooled DOR of 141.9 (95% CI 68.6–293.5), though the authors cautioned that "the risk of misdiagnosis remains considerable among studies enrolling clinical sepsis, as noninfectious conditions likely account for a certain proportion of cases, possibly leading to overestimation of presepsin accuracy." The findings suggest presepsin "was a robust biomarker" of EOS and warrant trials to assess its usefulness in guiding early empirical antibiotic treatment, especially for newborns born preterm.

Yoon et al. [128] performed the first systematic review and meta-analysis that evaluated the diagnostic value of presepsin for pediatric sepsis (not including neonates) and compare it with other biomarkers. A total of four studies [74, 129, 130] (one in Turkey, one in Egypt, and two in Slovakia) were published between 2016 and 2018. Three hundred eight patients (101 patients with sepsis, 127 non-sepsis patients, and 80 healthy volunteers) aged between 1 month and 18 years were included. The pooled diagnostic sensitivity of presepsin was 0.94 (95% confidence interval [CI]: 0.74–0.99,) specificity 0.71 (95% CI: 0.35–0.92), pooled DOR 32.87 (95% CI: 2.12–510.09), PLR 3.24 (95% CI, 1.14–12.38), and NLR 0.08 (95% CI, 0.01–0.74). Presepsin has higher sensitivity and diagnostic accuracy, but lower specificity, than PCT or CRP in detecting sepsis in children. The pooled sensitivity of presepsin (0.94) was higher than that of CRP (0.51) and PCT (0.76), whereas the overall specificity of presepsin (0.71) was lower than that of CRP (0.81) and PCT (0.76). The AUC of presepsin (0.925) was higher than that of CRP (0.715) and PCT (0.820). The high sensitivity of presepsin could be very useful for the exclusion of sepsis in pediatric patients when the level of this biomarker is normal or lower than the cut-off value. But, this result must be interpreted with caution, because the meta-analysis included only a few heterogeneous studies.

6.2 Presepsin as a prognostic marker

A growing body of literature indicates the potential of presepsin as a suitable biomarker for the assessment of severity, risk stratification especially for Gram-negative bacterial infection, the prognosis of sepsis and aid clinicians with the choice of appropriate treatment strategies at an early stage for optimal resource allocation. A change in presepsin levels may be an appropriate indicator for monitoring antibiotic therapy that improves the prognosis and increases the survival rate in severe sepsis or septic shock. Serial presepsin measurement can be used to evaluate changes in a patient's condition in the ICU. Patients with ≥50% decreased presepsin in ICU survived more than 90 days [131]. Reduction in presepsin levels on day 7 strongly correlates with the efficacy of antibiotic therapy [71]. The trend of presepsin decrease during serial prespsin measurement is a good prognostic sign, until an increase hints worse prognosis. The first few days in ICU are critical for the development of most severe complications, and elevated presepsin levels may be associated with the occurrence of severe sepsis complications and subsequent mortality in ICU. Shimoyama et al. [132] in the prospective cohort study, single-center ICU, with 83 patients reported that presepsin elevation upon ICU admission and on day 2 is a predictor of septic acute renal failure, presepsin on days 1 to 3 acute respiratory distress syndrome, presepsin on day 2 and Δ presepsin (day 2-day 1) for septic disseminated intravascular coagulation (DIC). Multivariate analysis revealed presepsin on day 2 to be a predictor of septic DIC. Combining presepsin with Glasgow Prognostic Score improved the specificity for predicting septic ARDS relative to using baseline presepsin values alone. The same authors [133] demonstrated that presepsin value on day 1 predicts 28-day mortality and death within 7 days of ICU admission.

In Hassan et al. [134] study, ICU patients with sepsis reported that presepsin levels within the first week had better prognostic accuracy than hsCRP in the prediction of sepsis-related in-hospital mortality. Patients who had higher levels of presepsin at admission than the cut-off value (>607 pg/ml) had a shortened survival period compared to patients who had lower levels. Klouche et al. [62] aimed to assess the prognostic value of presepsin in ICU patients with severe sepsis, septic shock, and severe community-acquired pneumonia. They identified presepsin levels that best predict ICU mortality in septic patients (1925 pg/ml), and those with community-acquired pneumonia at cutoff values (714 pg/ml). Kim et al. [135] performed a retrospective study included 157 septic patients (112 patients with sepsis; 45 patients with septic shock) admitted to ICU or ED, with the aim to explore the prognostic utilities of multi-marker approach using PCT, presepsin, galectin-3, and sST2 in septic patients for predicting 30-days mortality. Although the presepsin was higher in non-survivors compared with survivors, presepsin alone was not a significant predictor of 30-day mortality. But, the combination of presepsin with PCT, galectin-3, and soluble suppression of tumorigenicity-2 showed better performance in predicting 30-day all-cause mortality than the single use of presepsin for sepsis patients.

Drăgoescu et al. [136] in a recently published study assessed the efficacy of presepsin at admission in the prognosis of sepsis useful marker for prognosis of sepsis severity and mortality risk in 114 patients admitted to the ICU in comparison to CRP, erythrocyte sedimentation rate, white blood cells, and SOFA score. Presepsin values were significantly higher ($P < 0.001$) in patients with septic shock 2403 (1974–3278) ng/ml compared with those with sepsis 1476 (963–2413) ng/dl, as well as in non-survivors 2975 (2551–3647) ng/ml compared to survivors 1258 (963–1971) ng/dl. Presepsin levels higher than 1932 ng/ml had a sensitivity 79% and specificity 63% in predicting in-hospital mortality. The AUC was 0.726 (95% CI 0.635–0.806) ($P < 0.0001$), and it was significantly better than SOFA score, but similar to CRP in predicting sepsis severity. They also found that presepsin levels higher than 2365 ng/dl had a sensitivity 74% and specificity 88%. The AUC was 0.861 (95% CI 0.784–0.919) ($P < 0.0001$). Presepsin was a significantly better predictor of sepsis mortality than CRP, SOFA score.

In the study of Matera et al. [137] that included ICU patients with suspected sepsis, multivariate logistic regression analysis showed that only presepsin (within 6 h after admission) is an independent predictor of mortality, until PCT and CRP were not significant predictors.

Behnes et al. [44] evaluated the prognostic accuracy of presepsin in 116 patients with suspected severe sepsis or septic shock during the first week of ICU treatment.

Presepsin revealed a valuable diagnostic capacity to differentiate sepsis severity compared to other used biomarkers for sepsis such as PCT, IL-6, CRP, and WBC. Presepsin and IL-6 also showed prognostic value regarding 30 days and 6 months of all-cause mortality throughout the first week of ICU treatment. Multicenter prospective cohort study of Endo et al. [46] included 103 patients with sepsis admitted to the ED or ICU and compared the clinical utility of presepsin with other sepsis biomarkers including PCT, IL6, and CRP for evaluating the severity of sepsis during follow-up. Presepsin was the only biomarker that remained elevated after treatment application in the unfavorable prognosis group that had the most severe initial presentation and retained an association with an elevated risk of 28-day mortality during the follow-up period.

Presepsin was evaluated as a potential biomarker for bacterial infection relapse in critical care patients during hospitalization in ICU. In patients with a clinical recurrence of sepsis, presepsin levels remained high while PCT levels were normalized during the transient remission phase. The existence of high presepsin levels could alert clinicians to continue with antibiotic therapy in patients with sepsis [55].

Jovanovic et al. [138] evaluated the prognostic value of presepsin for ventilator-associated pneumonia (VAP) and sepsis in critically injured patients requiring mechanical ventilation and treatment in ICU. Presepsin levels were significantly higher in patients who developed VAP compared to those with SIRS and significantly higher in patients with sepsis compared to those with VAP or SIRS.

In the Multicenter Albumin Italian Outcome Sepsis (ALBIOS) [71], the first analysis included patients with severe sepsis or septic shock, and reported the median concentration of presepsin at ICU admission as 2269 (1171–4300) pg/ml in deceased patients, that was significantly higher than 1184 (875–2113) pg/ml in survived. Baseline presepsin was independently associated with the risk of ICU and 90-day mortality. Increasing concentrations of presepsin from day 1 to day 2 predicted higher ICU and 90-day mortality (adjusted $P < 0.0001$ and $P < 0.01$, respectively). The second analysis from the ALBIOS trial (enrolling patients with severe sepsis or septic shock in ICUs) [139] demonstrated that presepsin level was independently associated with the number and degree of organ dysfunctions or failures, coagulation disorders and ICU mortality. Provide the first evidence that presepsin measurements may have useful prognostic information for patients with severe sepsis or septic shock. Results showed that presepsin was the only variable independently associated with ICU and 28-day mortality. It also showed better prognostic accuracy than PCT in the range of SOFA score.

Two prospective cohort studies found that presepsin is an independent predictor of in-hospital mortality in a cohort of patients hospitalized due to sepsis [140] and in patients with sepsis-related ARDS [141]. Wen et al. [140] also found that the combination of presepsin elevation and SOFA score was a predictor of in-hospital mortality compared with a marker or stroke used alone. A recently published study by Aliu-Bejta et al. [142] in 2020 performed also in a cohort of hospitalized patients outside of ICU, found significantly higher baseline presepsin concentrations in patients with septic shock compared to septic patients (according to the sepsis-3 definition), especially in the first 72 h, confirming that presepsin concentrations had a good capacity for distinguishing disease severity. PCT and CRP levels did not differ significantly between the two severity groups.

A recently published single-center prospective observational study by Lee et al. [68] reported prognostic value of presepsin among patients with non-infectious organ failure, sepsis, and septic shock (in accordance with Sepsis-3 definition) in ED. They identified the most useful presepsin cut-off value (821 pg/ml) for the prediction of 30-day mortality among patients with sepsis and septic shock. Multivariate Cox proportional hazards model analyses of the 30-day mortality, identified presepsin as a significant predictor (HR 1.003; 95% CI 1.001–1.005; $P = 0.042$) together with lactate (HR 1.108; 95% CI 1.070–1.147; $P < 0.001$) and SOFA score (HR 1.264; 95% CI 1.167–1.369; $P < 0.001$).

Ulla et al. [60] reported that a higher level of presepsin at presentation in ED was correlated to 60-day mortality. Lu et al. [70] in 72 patients with sepsis in ED and 23 nonbacterial patients with SIRS reported presepsin's value as a prognostic marker of sepsis severity. They found that there was a significant difference in presepsin, among sepsis, severe sepsis, and septic shock group ($P < 0.05$). Statistically, a significant difference was noticed between the sepsis and severe sepsis group, as well as between the severe sepsis and septic shock group.

Presepsin may also retain significant predictive values in the ED, where initial evaluation may be a significant predictor of early mortality due to sepsis. The validity of presepsin as a prognostic marker of 30-day mortality in the ED was assessed in 123 patients with suspected infection in the ED and 123 healthy individuals [48]. Results showed that presepsin at admission had a similar outcome prediction as the clinical scores MEDS and APACHE II. The combination of presepsin with MEDS score improved the power for outcome prediction. Popa et al. [143] in a retrospective study of 95 patients with suspected infection in ED concluded that presepsin is an early marker of mortality in patients with sepsis. Ishikura et al. [97] evaluated 11 biomarkers in 82 patients with ≥1 SIRS criteria at admission to the ED, with the aim to define a biomarker panel to predict sepsis-induced DIC. The optimal panel was presepsin together with protein C is predictive of the severity of sepsis-induced DIC in suspected ED patients.

Three studies did not show so promising results about the relationship between presepsin and mortality. Enguix-Armada et al. [106] analyzed the prognostic value of CRP, PCT, presepsin mid-regional pro-adrenomedullin measured in the first 24 h from ICU admission. The outcome variables studied were 28-day mortality and length of stay in the ICU. The authors failed to detect any prognostic value presepsin measured in the first 24 h. Brodska et al. [144] in 30 consecutive patients admitted for sepsis to the mixed medical-surgical ICU, showed the opposite results, i.e., that presepsin did not outperform the traditional biomarkers (PCT, CRP, lactate) in mortality prognosis in critically ill patients with sepsis and SIRS. Koh et al. [145] evaluated the performance of presepsin as a biomarker for predicting in-hospital mortality in 153 patients with sepsis or sepsis shock admitted to ICU directly from ED. Although presepsin values were higher in the non-survivor compared to the survivor group, ROC analysis revealed poor performances of presepsin in predicting the prognosis of sepsis (AUC = 0.656, $P = 0.001$). Presepsin levels higher than 1176 pg/ml had a 66.7% sensitivity and 61.1% specificity in predicting in-hospital mortality.

The prognostic value of presepsin has also been evaluated in patients who are hospitalized with a known cause of infection. Two studies examined presepsin in confirmed pneumonia. Titova et al. [146] in 75 patients with pneumonia, sepsis, and other inflammatory diseases found that presepsin in patients with pneumogenic sepsis was higher compared to presepsin in patients with severe pneumonia and non-severe pneumonia. The high level of presepsin reflects the severity of pneumonia and the development of sepsis. Ugajin et al. [147] reported that presepsin levels on admission could be a useful predictor of 30-day mortality in hospitalized patients with pneumonia. Song et al. [148] examined if presepsin has some prognostic value in patients with enterocutaneous fistula and abdominal sepsis. Patients with higher presepsin levels had a more severe intra-abdominal infection, higher risks of complications, and failure of fistula closure compared with patients with low presepsin admission values group. Current evidence suggests that presepsin could be also a useful predictive marker for newly developing sepsis after abdominal surgery [149]. Prospective study by Bamba et al. [150] revealed that presepsin could also be a useful biomarker of sepsis secondary to fungal infections. Presepsin levels were increased in those patients with fungal bloodstream infection, with a positive association with the disease severity.

Presepsin has also been tested in an antimicrobial stewardship program. In a recent prospective, multicenter, not randomized trial from China Xiao et al. [151] compared presepsin guidance to control (standard of care) in sepsis. In the presepsin group, physicians were advised to stop the antibiotics by serum concentrations lower than 350 pg/ml or any baseline decrease of more than 80%. The antibiotic adjustment was encouraged when the blood presepsin concentration did not decline. Patients in the presepsin group had significantly ($P < 0.001$) more days without antibiotics [14.54 days (SD 9.01) compared with the control group 11.01 days (SD 7.73),]. Although the primary outcome (days without antibiotics at day 28) was achieved, mortality did not differ between treatment arms. Mortality in the presepsin group was not significantly different compared to control group at day 28 (17.7% vs. 18.2%; $P = 0.868$) and day 90 (19.9% vs. 19.5%; $P = 0.891$). Patients in the presepsin group had a significantly shorter hospital length of stay and lower healthcare costs compared with the control group.

6.2.1 *Systematic reviews and meta-analyses*

Two meta-analyses that evaluated the prognostic value of presepsin in adult septic patients have been recently published. The first of Yang et al. [152] included 10 studies [30, 42, 44, 48, 62, 135, 139, 153–155] with 1617 patients (580 non-survivors and 1037 survivors). Five out of ten included studies were conducted in ICU, three studies in ED, and six studies exclusively contained severe sepsis or septic shock. This is the first meta-analysis, that demonstrated that presepsin can predict mortality in patients with sepsis. Presepsin levels in samples taken within the first 24 h were significantly higher in non-survivors as compared to survivors: a weighted pooled SMD of 0.92 (0.62–1.22) for over-all mortality and 1.09 (0.78–1.41) for in-hospital or 30-days mortality ($P < 0.01$). In subgroups, divided by the sepsis severity or study site (ICU, ED), pooled SMD was consistently noting higher presepsin levels in non-survivals ($P < 0.05$).

Zhu et al. [156] further evaluate the relationship between presepsin and hospital mortality and provide additional information on pooled sensitivity and specificity to determine its prognostic performance. Nine publications [30, 42, 48, 135, 137, 139, 144, 154, 157], comprising 1561 patients, were included in this study. Since PCT was a widely used predictor of mortality, they performed a head-to-head comparison of presepsin and PCT in predicting all-cause mortality in these patients. The overall AUC of presepsin was 0.77 (95% CI, 0.73–0.81) with a pooled prognostic sensitivity 0.83 (95% CI, 0.72–0.90) and specificity 0.69 (95% CI, 0.63–0.74). Additionally, the PLR, NLR, and DOR of presepsin were 2.6 (95% CI, 2.1–3.3), 0.25 (95% CI, 0.15–0.44), and 10 (95% CI, 5–22), respectively. It was found that there is no statistically significant difference between presepsin and PCT, implying that both predictors are promising prognostic biomarkers of sepsis.

7. Conclusions

Within the last decade, a broad range of molecular biomarkers for sepsis has been reported. One of the most promising emerging biomarkers is presepsin, gaining relevance year by year. After the initial report in 2005, a strong body of literature comprised of more than 280 clinical studies, systematic reviews, and meta-analyses, indicated that presepsin could be used as a relevant routine daily clinical tool for early diagnosis, risk stratification, and predicting clinical progression, short-term and long-term outcomes, and guiding therapeutic management in adult, neonates, and pediatric sepsis patient. That presepsin is still a marker in focus, is shown by the fact that almost 70% of studies were published in the last 5 years. With the change of sepsis definition in Sepsis-3, the utility of presepsin is currently being reevaluated, with consistently encouraging results. In addition, presepsin concentration can now be routinely measured in whole blood, in approximately 15 min, using point-of-care devices in different clinical settings (ED, ICU). A potential advantage of presepsin resides in the possibility of its measuring in non-invasive biological fluids such as urine, saliva, as well as tracheal aspirate for adults, children, and infants.

Despite presepsin represents a promising biomarker, it still faces numerous challenges and criticisms that require further elucidation. The studies in favor of the use of presepsin are heterogenous in the sense they use the sepsis-2 definition, and examine clinically heterogenic patient groups at risk of sepsis in a variety of different settings, with the small sample size as a common limitation.

Inter-assay disagreement can represent a confounding factor in the interpretation of test results in different studies. The definition of an optimal cut-off is very important. Instead of using static threshold presepsin concentrations, serial monitoring of presepsin levels would prove more helpful to clinicians to follow an individual patient's response to therapy. Further prospective studies with larger and more diverse populations are required to establish the presepsin cut-off for the diagnosis and prognosis of infections. Consensus regarding time sampling strategy in infants is particularly of great importance. Also, conversion of presepsin level from pg/ml to multiple medians as measurement units will be more than justified in the assessment of perinatal sepsis. Studies that evaluated the impact of presepsin on therapeutic decisions are still limited. Specifically designed randomized clinical trials are needed to determine the usefulness and safety of early measurement of presepsin to guide early empirical antibiotic treatment, particularly in preterm newborns. Will presepsin be incorporated in antimicrobial stewardship programs that will contribute to reducing antimicrobial overuse in septic patients without compromising the clinical outcome, remains to be seen. Although, current evidence on biomarkers and pharmacokinetic optimization of antibiotics in critically ill patients is limited, maybe in the future, presepsin-based drug monitoring for dose optimization will be proposed.

As it has already been touched on in the chapter, in some clinical conditions (renal failure, burns, etc.), presepsin levels can be altered in the absence of sepsis. Presepsin levels may be higher in some physiological conditions like in preterm newborns and advanced age patients, in which concentrations reach the threshold at which the diagnosis of sepsis would be highly suspected in human beings. Presepsin is also affected by the translocation of intestinal microbial flora. Future studies are necessary, for the identification of these conditions and the determination of appropriate cut-off values based on age and associated diseases.

Many studies in different clinical settings that compared the diagnostic and prognostic efficacy of presepsin with CRP and/or PCT, reported controversial results. Presepsin does not appear to be clearly superior to the biomarkers commonly used in the assessment of sepsis, although mainly performances place presepsin at the level of PCT. Compared to PCT, the significance of presepsin elevation is easy to understand, as it results from a dose–response mechanism of the host-pathogen interaction. Presepsin increases with every type of bacteria and fungi. In neonatal sepsis, presepsin compared to PCT is more effective in diagnosing and guiding therapy.

The combination of presepsin with traditional sepsis biomarkers CRP and/or PCT, or with other novel biomarkers (triggering receptor expressed on myeloid cells-1, neutrophil cluster of differentiation-64, soluble urokinase-type plasminogen activator receptor, mid-regional pro-adrenomedullin, cell-free DNA, microRNAs, interleukin-27, etc) into a bio-score, together with physician expertise and clinical judgment, may be particularly useful in the diagnosis of sepsis or the risk stratification of patients with sepsis. High-quality prospective studies with larger, diverse populations with an eye on specific subgroups are more than warranted. It seems that presepsin merits further study to delineate its specific area of utility.

Conflict of interest

The author declares no conflict of interest.

Author details

Sanja Stankovic[1,2]

1 Center for Medical Biochemistry, University Clinical Center of Serbia, Belgrade, Serbia

2 Faculty of Medical Sciences, University of Kragujevac, Kragujevac, Serbia

*Address all correspondence to: sanjast2013@gmail.com

References

[1] Singer M, Deutschman CS, Seymour CW, Shankar-Hari M, Annane D, Bauer M, et al. The third international consensus definitions for Sepsis and septic shock (sepsis-3). Journal of the American Medical Association. 2016;**315**(8):801-810. DOI: 10.1001/jama.2016.0287

[2] Shane AL, Sánchez PJ, Stoll BJ. Neonatal sepsis. Lancet. 2017;**390**(10104):1770-1780. DOI: 10.1016/S0140-6736(17)31002-4

[3] Fleischmann C, Scherag A, Adhikari NK, Hartog CS, Tsaganos T, Schlattmann P, et al. International forum of acute care trialists. Assessment of global incidence and mortality of hospital-treated sepsis. Current estimates and limitations. American Journal of Respiratory and Critical Care Medicine. 2016;**193**(3):259-272. DOI: 10.1164/rccm.201504-0781OC

[4] Rudd KE, Johnson SC, Agesa KM, Shackelford KA, Tsoi D, Kievlan DR, et al. Global, regional, and national sepsis incidence and mortality, 1990-2017: Analysis for the global burden of disease study. Lancet. 2020;**395**(10219):200-211. DOI: 10.1016/S0140-6736(19)32989-7

[5] World Health Organization. Global Report on the Epidemiology and Burden of Sepsis: Current Evidence, Identifying Gaps and Future Directions. Geneva, Switzerland: World Health Organization; 2020. Available from: https://apps.who.int/iris/handle/10665/334216. License: CC BY-NC-SA 3.0 IGO

[6] Fleischmann-Struzek C, Goldfarb DM, Schlattmann P, Schlapbach LJ, Reinhart K, Kissoon N. The global burden of paediatric and neonatal sepsis: A systematic review. The Lancet Respiratory Medicine. 2018;**6**(3):223-230. DOI: 10.1016/S2213-2600(18)30063-8

[7] Seymour CW, Gesten F, Prescott HC, Friedrich ME, Iwashyna TJ, Phillips GS, et al. Time to treatment and mortality during mandated emergency care for sepsis. The New England Journal of Medicine. 2017;**376**(23):2235-2244. DOI: 10.1056/NEJMoa1703058

[8] Paoli CJ, Reynolds MA, Sinha M, Gitlin M, Crouser E. Epidemiology and costs of sepsis in the United States-an analysis based on timing of diagnosis and severity level. Critical Care Medicine. 2018;**46**(12):1889-1897. DOI: 10.1097/CCM.0000000000003342

[9] Cervellin G, Schuetz P, Lippi G. Toward a holistic approach for diagnosing sepsis in the emergency department. Advances in Clinical Chemistry. 2019;**92**:201-216. DOI: 10.1016/bs.acc.2019.04.004

[10] Lippi G. Sepsis biomarkers: Past, present and future. Clinical Chemistry and Laboratory Medicine. 2019;**57**(9):1281-1283. DOI: 10.1515/cclm-2018-1347

[11] Barichello T, Generoso JS, Singer M, Dal-Pizzol F. Biomarkers for sepsis: More than just fever and leukocytosis-a narrative review. Critical Care. 2022;**26**(1):14. DOI: 10.1186/s13054-021-03862-5

[12] Schenz J, Weigand MA, Uhle F. Molecular and biomarker-based diagnostics in early sepsis: Current challenges and future perspectives. Expert Review of Molecular Diagnostics. 2019;**19**(12):1069-1078. DOI: 10.1080/14737159.2020.1680285

[13] Lodise TP, McKinnon PS, Swiderski L, Rybak MJ. Outcomes

analysis of delayed antibiotic treatment for hospital-acquired *Staphylococcus aureus* bacteremia. Clinical Infectious Diseases. 2003;**36**(11):1418-1423. DOI: 10.1086/375057

[14] Pruinelli L, Westra BL, Yadav P, Hoff A, Steinbach M, Kumar V, et al. Delay within the 3-hour surviving sepsis campaign guideline on mortality for patients with severe sepsis and septic shock. Critical Care Medicine. 2018;**46**(4):500-505. DOI: 10.1097/CCM.0000000000002949

[15] Opal SM, Wittebole X. Biomarkers of infection and sepsis. Critical Care Clinics. 2020;**36**(1):11-22. DOI: 10.1016/j.ccc.2019.08.002

[16] Pierrakos C, Velissaris D, Bisdorff M, Marshall JC, Vincent JL. Biomarkers of sepsis: Time for a reappraisal. Critical Care. 2020;**24**(1):287. DOI: 10.1186/s13054-020-02993-5

[17] Strimbu K, Tavel JA. What are biomarkers? Current Opinion in HIV and AIDS. 2010;**5**(6):463-466. DOI: 10.1097/COH.0b013e32833ed177

[18] Rhodes A, Evans LE, Alhazzani W, Levy MM, Antonelli M, Ferrer R, et al. Surviving Sepsis campaign: International guidelines for management of sepsis and septic shock: 2016. Critical Care Medicine. 2017;**45**(3):486-552. DOI: 10.1097/CCM.0000000000002255

[19] Lippi G, Cervellin G. Can presepsin be used for screening invasive fungal infections? The Annals of Translational Medicine. 2019;**7**(5):87. DOI: 10.21037/atm.2019.01.40

[20] Chenevier-Gobeaux C, Borderie D, Weiss N, Mallet-Coste T, Claessens YE. Presepsin (sCD14-ST), an innate immune response marker in sepsis. Clinica Chimica Acta. 2015;**450**:97-103. DOI: 10.1016/j.cca.2015.06.026

[21] Wright SD, Ramos RA, Tobias PS, Ulevitch RJ, Mathison JC. CD14, a receptor for complexes of lipopolysaccharide (LPS) and LPS binding protein. Science. 1990;**249**(4975):1431-1433. DOI: 10.1126/science.1698311

[22] Jack RS, Fan X, Bernheiden M, Rune G, Ehlers M, Weber A, et al. Lipopolysaccharide-binding protein is required to combat a murine gram-negative bacterial infection. Nature. 1997;**389**(6652):742-745. DOI: 10.1038/39622

[23] Ferrero E, Goyert SM. Nucleotide sequence of the gene encoding the monocyte differentiation antigen, CD14. Nucleic Acids Research. 1988;**16**(9):4173. DOI: 10.1093/nar/16.9.4173

[24] Haziot A, Chen S, Ferrero E, Low MG, Silber R, Goyert SM. The monocyte differentiation antigen, CD14, is anchored to the cell membrane by a phosphatidylinositol linkage. Journal of Immunology. 1988;**141**(2):547-552 PMID: 3385210

[25] Azim A. Presepsin: A promising biomarker for sepsis. Indian Journal of Critical Care Medicine. 2021;**25**(2):117-118. DOI: 10.5005/jp-journals-10071-23741

[26] Le-Barillec K, Si-Tahar M, Balloy V, Chignard M. Proteolysis of monocyte CD14 by human leukocyte elastase inhibits lipopolysaccharide-mediated cell activation. The Journal of Clinical Investigation. 1999;**103**(7):1039-1046. DOI: 10.1172/JCI5779

[27] Labeta MO, Durieux JJ, Fernandez N, Herrmann R, Ferrara P. Release from a human monocyte-like cell line of two different soluble forms of the lipopolysaccharide receptor, CD14. European Journal of Immunology. 1993;**23**(9):2144-2151. DOI: 10.1002/eji.1830230915

[28] Bowyer JF, Sarkar S, Burks SM, Hess JN, Tolani S, O'Callaghan JP, et al. Microglial activation and responses to vasculature that result from an acute LPS exposure. Neurotoxicology. 2020;**77**:181-192. DOI: 10.1016/j.neuro.2020.01.014

[29] Zanoni I, Ostuni R, Marek LR, Barresi S, Barbalat R, Barton GM, et al. CD14 controls the LPS-induced endocytosis of toll-like receptor 4. Cell. 2011;**147**(4):868-880. DOI: 10.1016/j.cell.2011.09.051

[30] Ali FT, Ali MA, Elnakeeb MM, Bendary HN. Presepsin is an early monitoring biomarker for predicting clinical outcome in patients with sepsis. Clinica Chimica Acta. 2016;(460):93-101. DOI: 10.1016/j.cca.2016.06.030

[31] Nakamura M, Takeuchi T, Naito K, Shirakawa K, Hosaka Y, Yamasaki F, et al. Early elevation of plasma soluble CD14 subtype, a novel biomarker for sepsis, in a rabbit cecal ligation and puncture model. Critical Care. 2008;**12**(Suppl 2):P194. DOI: 10.1186/cc6415

[32] Chenevier-Gobeaux C, Bardet V, Poupet H, Poyart C, Borderie D, Claessens YE. Presepsin (sCD14-ST) secretion and kinetics by peripheral blood mononuclear cells and monocytic THP-1 cell line. Annales de Biologie Clinique (Paris). 2016;**74**(1):93-97. DOI: 10.1684/abc.2015.1112

[33] Shirakawa K, Naitou K, Hirose J, Takahashi T, Furusako S. Presepsin (sCD14-ST): Development and evaluation of one-step ELISA with a new standard that is similar to the form of presepsin in septic patients. Clinical Chemistry and Laboratory Medicine. 2011;**49**(5):937-939. DOI: 10.1515/CCLM.2011.145

[34] Ward G, Simpson A, Boscato L, Hickman PE. The investigation of interferences in immunoassay. Clinical Biochemistry. 2017;**50**(18):1306-1311. DOI: 10.1016/j.clinbiochem.2017.08.015

[35] Okamura Y, Yokoi H. Development of a point-of-care assay system for measurement of presepsin (sCD14-ST). Clinica Chimica Acta. 2011;**412**(23-24):2157-2161. DOI: 10.1016/j.cca.2011.07.024

[36] Available from: https://www.accessdata.fda.gov/cdrh_docs/reviews/K100130.pdf [Accessed: 01 August 2022].

[37] Yaegashi Y, Shirakawa K, Sato N, Suzuki Y, Kojika M, Imai S, et al. Evaluation of a newly identified soluble CD14 subtype as a marker for sepsis. Journal of Infection and Chemotherapy. 2005;**11**(5):234-238. DOI: 10.1007/s10156-005-0400-4

[38] Kang T, Yoo J, Choi H, Lee S, Jekarl DW, Kim Y. Performance evaluation of presepsin using a Sysmex HISCL-5000 analyzer and determination of reference interval. Journal of Clinical Laboratory Analysis. 2022;**36**(9):e24618. DOI: 10.1002/jcla.24618

[39] Galliera E, Massaccesi L, Yu L, He J, Ranucci M, Corsi Romanelli MM. SCD14-ST and new generation inflammatory biomarkers in the prediction of COVID-19 outcome. Biomolecules. 2022;**12**(6):826. DOI: 10.3390/biom12060826

[40] Shozushima T, Takahashi G, Matsumoto N, Kojika M, Okamura Y, Endo S. Usefulness of presepsin (sCD14-ST) measurements as a marker for the diagnosis and severity of sepsis that satisfied diagnostic criteria of systemic inflammatory response syndrome. Journal of Infection and Chemotherapy. 2011;**17**(6):764-769. DOI: 10.1007/s10156-011-0254-x

[41] Claessens YE, Trabattoni E, Grabar S, Quinquis L, Der Sahakian G, Anselmo M, et al. Plasmatic presepsin (sCD14-ST) concentrations in acute pyelonephritis in adult patients. Clinica Chimica Acta. 2017;**464**:182-188. DOI: 10.1016/j.cca.2016.11.036

[42] Liu B, Chen YX, Yin Q, Zhao YZ, Li CS. Diagnostic value and prognostic evaluation of presepsin for sepsis in an emergency department. Critical Care. 2013;**17**(5):R244. DOI: 10.1186/cc13070

[43] Chenevier-Gobeaux C, Trabattoni E, Roelens M, Borderie D, Claessens YE. Presepsin (sCD14-ST) in emergency department: The need for adapted threshold values? Clinica Chimica Acta. 2014;**427**:34-36. DOI: 10.1016/j.cca.2013.09.019

[44] Behnes M, Bertsch T, Lepiorz D, Lang S, Trinkmann F, Brueckmann M, et al. Diagnostic and prognostic utility of soluble CD 14 subtype (presepsin) for severe sepsis and septic shock during the first week of intensive care treatment. Critical Care. 2014;**18**(5):507. DOI: 10.1186/s13054-014-0507-z

[45] Kweon OJ, Choi JH, Park SK, Park AJ. Usefulness of presepsin (sCD14 subtype) measurements as a new marker for the diagnosis and prediction of disease severity of sepsis in the Korean population. Journal of Critical Care. 2014;**29**(6):965-970. DOI: 10.1016/j.jcrc.2014.06.014

[46] Endo S, Suzuki Y, Takahashi G, Shozushima T, Ishikura H, Murai A, et al. Usefulness of presepsin in the diagnosis of sepsis in a multicenter prospective study. Journal of Infection and Chemotherapy. 2012;**18**(6):891-897. DOI: 10.1007/s10156-012-0435-2

[47] Giavarina D, Carta M. Determination of reference interval for presepsin, an early marker for sepsis. Biochemia Medica (Zagreb). 2015;**25**(1):64-68. DOI: 10.11613/BM.2015.007

[48] Carpio R, Zapata J, Spanuth E, Hess G. Utility of presepsin (sCD14-ST) as a diagnostic and prognostic marker of sepsis in the emergency department. Clinica Chimica Acta. 2015;**450**:169-175. DOI: 10.1016/j.cca.2015.08.013

[49] Mussap M, Puxeddu E, Burrai P, Noto A, Cibecchini F, Testa M, et al. Soluble CD14 subtype (sCD14-ST) presepsin in critically ill preterm newborns: Preliminary reference ranges. The Journal of Maternal-Fetal & Neonatal Medicine. 2012;**25**(Suppl 5):51-53. DOI: 10.3109/14767058.2012.717462

[50] Pugni L, Pietrasanta C, Milani S, Vener C, Ronchi A, Falbo M, et al. Presepsin (soluble CD14 subtype): Reference ranges of a new sepsis marker in term and preterm neonates. PLoS One. 2015;**10**(12):e0146020. DOI: 10.1371/journal.pone.0146020

[51] Poggi C, Vasarri MV, Boni L, Pugni L, Mosca F, Dani C. Reference ranges of presepsin in preterm infants in the first 48 h of life: A multicenter observational study. Clinica Chimica Acta. 2020;**508**:191-196. DOI: 10.1016/j.cca.2020.05.040

[52] Nur Ergor S, Yalaz M, Altun Koroglu O, Sozmen E, Akisu M, Kultursay N. Reference ranges of presepsin (soluble CD14 subtype) in term and preterm neonates without infection, in relation to gestational and postnatal age, in the first 28 days of life. Clinical Biochemistry. 2020;**77**:7-13. DOI: 10.1016/j.clinbiochem.2019.12.007

[53] Kollmann TR, Levy O, Montgomery RR, Goriely S. Innate immune function by toll-like receptors: Distinct responses in newborns and the

elderly. Immunity. 2012;**37**(5):771-783. DOI: 10.1016/j.immuni.2012.10.014

[54] Nagata T, Yasuda Y, Ando M, Abe T, Katsuno T, Kato S, et al. Clinical impact of kidney function on presepsin levels. PLoS One. 2015;**10**(6):e0129159. DOI: 10.1371/journal.pone.0129159

[55] Sargentini V, Ceccarelli G, D'Alessandro M, Collepardo D, Morelli A, D'Egidio A, et al. Presepsin as a potential marker for bacterial infection relapse in critical care patients. A preliminary study. Clinical Chemistry and Laboratory Medicine. 2015;**53**(4):567-573. DOI: 10.1515/cclm-2014-0119

[56] Lin J, Sun H, Li J, Zheng Y, Shao C, Zhang YH, et al. Role of presepsin for the assessment of acute cholangitis severity. Clinical Laboratory. 2016;**62**(4):679-687. DOI: 10.7754/clin.lab.2015.150832

[57] Tsuchida T, Ie K, Okuse C, Hirose M, Nishisako H, Torikai K, et al. Determining the factors affecting serum presepsin level and its diagnostic utility: A cross-sectional study. Journal of Infection and Chemotherapy. 2021;**27**(4):585-591. DOI: 10.1016/j.jiac.2020.11.013

[58] de Guadiana Romualdo LG, Torrella PE, Acebes SR, Otón MDA, Sánchez RJ, Holgado AH, et al. Diagnostic accuracy of presepsin (sCD14-ST) as a biomarker of infection and sepsis in the emergency department. Clinica Chimica Acta. 2017;**464**:6-11. DOI: 10.1016/j.cca.2016.11.003

[59] Romualdo LG, Torrella PE, González MV, Sánchez RJ, Holgado AH, Freire AO, et al. Diagnostic accuracy of presepsin (soluble CD14 subtype) for prediction of bacteremia in patients with systemic inflammatory response syndrome in the emergency department. Clinical Biochemistry. 2014;**47**(7-8):505-508. DOI: 10.1016/j.clinbiochem.2014.02.011

[60] Ulla M, Pizzolato E, Lucchiari M, Loiacono M, Soardo F, Forno D, et al. Diagnostic and prognostic value of presepsin in the management of sepsis in the emergency department: A multicenter prospective study. Critical Care. 2013;**17**(4):R168. DOI: 10.1186/cc12847

[61] Cakır Madenci Ö, Yakupoğlu S, Benzonana N, Yücel N, Akbaba D, Orçun KA. Evaluation of soluble CD14 subtype (presepsin) in burn sepsis. Burns. 2014;**40**(4):664-669. DOI: 10.1016/j.burns.2013.08.024

[62] Klouche K, Cristol JP, Devin J, Gilles V, Kuster N, Larcher R, et al. Diagnostic and prognostic value of soluble CD14 subtype (Presepsin) for sepsis and community-acquired pneumonia in ICU patients. Annals of Intensive Care. 2016;**6**(1):59. DOI: 10.1186/s13613-016-0160-6

[63] Vodnik T, Kaljevic G, Tadic T, Majkic-Singh N. Presepsin (sCD14-ST) in preoperative diagnosis of abdominal sepsis. Clinical Chemistry and Laboratory Medicine. 2013;**51**(10):2053-2062. DOI: 10.1515/cclm-2013-0061

[64] Hou YS, Wang H, Chen H, Wu LF, Lu LF, He Y. Pathfast presepsin assay for early diagnosis of systemic inflammatory response syndrome in patients with nephrolithiasis. BioMed Research International. 2015;**2015**:792572. DOI: 10.1155/2015/792572

[65] Godnic M, Stubljar D, Skvarc M, Jukic T. Diagnostic and prognostic value of sCD14-ST--presepsin for patients admitted to hospital intensive care unit (ICU). Wiener Klinische Wochenschrift. 2015;**127**(13-14):521-527. DOI: 10.1007/s00508-015-0719-5

[66] Leli C, Ferranti M, Marrano U, Al Dhahab ZS, Bozza S, Cenci E, et al. Diagnostic accuracy of presepsin (sCD14-ST) and procalcitonin for prediction of bacteraemia and bacterial DNAaemia in patients with suspected sepsis. Journal of Medical Microbiology. 2016;**65**(8):713-719. DOI: 10.1099/jmm.0.000278

[67] Contenti J, Occelli C, Lemoel F, Ferrari P, Levraut J. Presepsin versus other biomarkers to predict sepsis and septic shock in patients with infection defined by Sepsis-3 criteria: The PREDI study of diagnostic accuracy. Emergencias. 2019;**31**(5):311-317 PMID: 31625302

[68] Lee S, Song J, Park DW, Seok H, Ahn S, Kim J, et al. Diagnostic and prognostic value of presepsin and procalcitonin in non-infectious organ failure, sepsis, and septic shock: A prospective observational study according to the Sepsis-3 definitions. BMC Infectious Diseases. 2022;**22**(1):8. DOI: 10.1186/s12879-021-07012-8

[69] Sargentini V, Collepardo D, Alessandro D, Petralito M, Ceccarelli G, Alessandri F, et al. Role of biomarkers in adult sepsis and their application for a good laboratory practice: A pilot study. Journal of Biological Regulators and Homeostatic Agents. 2017;**31**(4):1147-1154 PMID: 29254328

[70] Lu B, Zhang Y, Li C, Liu C, Yao Y, Su M, et al. The utility of presepsin in diagnosis and risk stratification for the emergency patients with sepsis. The American Journal of Emergency Medicine. 2018;**36**(8):1341-1345. DOI: 10.1016/j.ajem.2017.12.038

[71] Masson S, Caironi P, Fanizza C, Thomae R, Bernasconi R, Noto A, et al. Circulating presepsin (soluble CD14 subtype) as a marker of host response in patients with severe sepsis or septic shock: Data from the multicenter, randomized ALBIOS trial. Intensive Care Medicine. 2015;**41**(1):12-20. DOI: 10.1007/s00134-014-3514-2

[72] Stoma I, Karpov I, Uss A, Rummo O, Milanovich N, Iskrov I. Diagnostic value of sepsis biomarkers in hematopoietic stem cell transplant recipients in a condition of high prevalence of gram-negative pathogens. Hematology/Oncology and Stem Cell Therapy. 2017;**10**(1):15-21. DOI: 10.1016/j.hemonc.2016.09.002

[73] Stoma I, Karpov I, Uss A, Krivenko S, Iskrov I, Milanovich N, et al. Combination of sepsis biomarkers may indicate an invasive fungal infection in haematological patients. Biomarkers. 2019;**24**(4):401-406. DOI: 10.1080/1354750X.2019.1600023

[74] Plesko M, Suvada J, Makohusova M, Waczulikova I, Behulova D, Vasilenkova A, et al. The role of CRP, PCT, IL-6 and presepsin in early diagnosis of bacterial infectious complications in paediatric haemato-oncological patients. Neoplasma. 2016;**63**(5):752-760. DOI: 10.4149/neo_2016_512

[75] Chen M, Zhu Y. Utility of sTREM-1 and presepsin (sCD14-ST) as diagnostic and prognostic markers of sepsis. Clinical Laboratory. 2020;**66**(4). DOI: 10.7754/Clin.Lab.2019.190508

[76] Ruangsomboon O, Panjaikaew P, Monsomboon A, Chakorn T, Permpikul C, Limsuwat C. Diagnostic and prognostic utility of presepsin for sepsis in very elderly patients in the emergency department. Clinica Chimica Acta. 2020;**510**:723-732. DOI: 10.1016/j.cca.2020.09.014

[77] Botondi V, D'Adamo E, Plebani M, Trubiani O, Perrotta M, Di Ricco L,

et al. Perinatal presepsin assessment: A new sepsis diagnostic tool? Clinical Chemistry and Laboratory Medicine. 2022;**60**(8):1136-1144. DOI: 10.1515/cclm-2022-0277

[78] Chen L, Xiao T, Luo Y, Qiu Q, Que R, Huang X, et al. Soluble CD14 subtype (sCD14-ST) is a biomarker for neonatal sepsis. International Journal of Clinical and Experimental Pathology. 2017;**10**(9):9718-9724

[79] Gad GI, Shinkar DM, Kamel El-Din MM, Nagi HM. The utility of soluble CD14 subtype in early diagnosis of culture-proven early-onset neonatal sepsis and prediction of outcome. American Journal of Perinatology. 2020;**37**(5):497-502. DOI: 10.1055/s-0039-1683863

[80] Mussap M, Puxeddu E, Puddu M, Ottonello G, Coghe F, Comite P, et al. Soluble CD14 subtype (sCD14-ST) presepsin in premature and full term critically ill newborns with sepsis and SIRS. Clinica Chimica Acta. 2015;**451**(Pt A):65-70. DOI: 10.1016/j.cca.2015.07.025

[81] Kamel M, Abd-ullah H, El Sayed M, Abdel AR. Presepsin as an early predictor of neonatal sepsis. International Journal of Pediatrics. 2021;**9**(4):13359-13369. DOI: 10.22038/IJP.2021.55127.4345

[82] Değirmencioğlu H, Ozer Bekmez B, Derme T, Öncel MY, Canpolat FE, Tayman C. Presepsin and fetuin-a dyad for the diagnosis of proven sepsis in preterm neonates. BMC Infectious Diseases. 2019;**19**(1):695. DOI: 10.1186/s12879-019-4316-5

[83] Miyosawa Y, Akazawa Y, Kamiya M, Nakamura C, Takeuchi Y, Kusakari M, et al. Presepsin as a predictor of positive blood culture in suspected neonatal sepsis. Pediatrics International. 2018;**60**(2):157-161. DOI: 10.1111/ped.13469

[84] Montaldo P, Rosso R, Santantonio A, Chello G, Giliberti P. Presepsin for the detection of early-onset sepsis in preterm newborns. Pediatric Research. 2017;**81**(2):329-334. DOI: 10.1038/pr.2016.217

[85] Topcuoglu S, Arslanbuga C, Gursoy T, Aktas A, Karatekin G, Uluhan R, et al. Role of presepsin in the diagnosis of late-onset neonatal sepsis in preterm infants. The Journal of Maternal-Fetal & Neonatal Medicine. 2016;**29**(11):1834-1839. DOI: 10.3109/14767058.2015.1064885

[86] Hashem HE, Abdel Halim RM, El Masry SA, Mokhtar AM, Abdelaal NM. The utility of neutrophil CD64 and presepsin as diagnostic, prognostic, and monitoring biomarkers in neonatal sepsis. International Journal of Microbiology. 2020;**2020**:8814892. DOI: 10.1155/2020/8814892

[87] Ozdemir AA, Elgormus Y. Diagnostic value of presepsin in detection of early-onset neonatal sepsis. American Journal of Perinatology. 2017;**34**(6):550-556. DOI: 10.1055/s-0036-1593851

[88] Sabry JH, Elfeky OA, Elsadek AE, Eldaly AA. Presepsin as an early reliable diagnostic and prognostic marker of neonatal sepsis. International Journal of Advanced Research. 2016;**6**:1538-1549

[89] Pietrasanta C, Ronchi A, Vener C, Poggi C, Ballerini C, Testa L, et al. Presepsin (soluble CD14 subtype) as an early marker of neonatal sepsis and septic shock: A prospective diagnostic trial. Antibiotics (Basel). 2021;**10**(5):580. DOI: 10.3390/antibiotics10050580

[90] Poggi C, Bianconi T, Gozzini E, Generoso M, Dani C. Presepsin for the

detection of late-onset sepsis in preterm newborns. Pediatrics. 2015;**135**(1):68-75. DOI: 10.1542/peds.2014-1755

[91] Zhang J, Hu ZD, Song J, Shao J. Diagnostic value of presepsin for sepsis: A systematic review and meta-analysis. Medicine (Baltimore). 2015;**94**(47):e2158. DOI: 10.1097/MD.0000000000002158

[92] Nakamura Y, Ishikura H, Nishida T, Kawano Y, Yuge R, Ichiki R, et al. Usefulness of presepsin in the diagnosis of sepsis in patients with or without acute kidney injury. BMC Anesthesiology. 2014;**14**:88. DOI: 10.1186/1471-2253-14-88

[93] Wu J, Hu L, Zhang G, Wu F, He T. Accuracy of presepsin in sepsis diagnosis: A systematic review and meta-analysis. PLoS One. 2015;**10**(7):e0133057. DOI: 10.1371/journal.pone.0133057

[94] Su MH, Shou ST. Prognostic value of presepsin for diagnosis and severity assessment of sepsis. Chinese Journal of Clinical Laboratory Science. 2014;**2**:106-108 +111

[95] Yu J, Shao Q, Wang Q, Zhang XH, Huang K. Combined determination of presepsin, procalcitonin and C reactive protein for early diagnosis and prognostic assessment of severe trauma patients with sepsis. Chinese Journal of Clinical Laboratory Science. 2014;**3**:200-203

[96] Zhang X, Liu D, Liu YN, Wang R, Xie LX. The accuracy of presepsin (sCD14-ST) for the diagnosis of sepsis in adults: A meta-analysis. Critical Care. 2015;**19**(1):323. DOI: 10.1186/s13054-015-1032-4

[97] Ishikura H, Nishida T, Murai A, Nakamura Y, Irie Y, Tanaka J, et al. New diagnostic strategy for sepsis-induced disseminated intravascular coagulation: A prospective single-center observational study. Critical Care. 2014;**18**(1):R19. DOI: 10.1186/cc13700

[98] Zheng Z, Jiang L, Ye L, Gao Y, Tang L, Zhang M. The accuracy of presepsin for the diagnosis of sepsis from SIRS: A systematic review and meta-analysis. Annals of Intensive Care. 2015;**5**(1):48. DOI: 10.1186/s13613-015-0089-1

[99] Tong X, Cao Y, Yu M, Han C. Presepsin as a diagnostic marker for sepsis: Evidence from a bivariate meta-analysis. Therapeutics and Clinical Risk Management. 2015;(11):1027-1033. DOI: 10.2147/TCRM.S84811

[100] Takahashi G, Shibata S, Ishikura H, Miura M, Fukui Y, Inoue Y, et al. Presepsin in the prognosis of infectious diseases and diagnosis of infectious disseminated intravascular coagulation: A prospective, multicentre, observational study. European Journal of Anaesthesiology. 2015;**32**(3):199-206. DOI: 10.1097/EJA.0000000000000178

[101] Liu Y, Hou JH, Li Q, Chen KJ, Wang SN, Wang JM. Biomarkers for diagnosis of sepsis in patients with systemic inflammatory response syndrome: A systematic review and meta-analysis. Springerplus. 2016;**5**(1):2091. DOI: 10.1186/s40064-016-3591-5

[102] Wu CC, Lan HM, Han ST, Chaou CH, Yeh CF, Liu SH, et al. Comparison of diagnostic accuracy in sepsis between presepsin, procalcitonin, and C-reactive protein: A systematic review and meta-analysis. Annals of Intensive Care. 2017;**7**(1):91. DOI: 10.1186/s13613-017-0316-z

[103] Brenner T, Fleming T, Uhle F, Silaff S, Schmitt F, Salgado E, et al. Methylglyoxal as a new biomarker in patients with septic shock: An

observational clinical study. Critical Care. 2014;**18**(6):683. DOI: 10.1186/s13054-014-0683-x

[104] Hayashida K, Kondo Y, Hara Y, Aihara M, Yamakawa K. Head-to-head comparison of procalcitonin and presepsin for the diagnosis of sepsis in critically ill adult patients: A protocol for a systematic review and meta-analysis. BMJ Open. 2017;**7**(3):e014305. DOI: 10.1136/bmjopen-2016-014305

[105] Kondo Y, Umemura Y, Hayashida K, Hara Y, Aihara M, Yamakawa K. Diagnostic value of procalcitonin and presepsin for sepsis in critically ill adult patients: A systematic review and meta-analysis. Journal of Intensive Care. 2019;**7**:22. DOI: 10.1186/s40560-019-0374-4

[106] Enguix-Armada A, Escobar-Conesa R, García-De La Torre A. De La Torre-Prados MV. Usefulness of several biomarkers in the management of septic patients: C-reactive protein, procalcitonin, presepsin and mid-regional pro-adrenomedullin. Clinical Chemistry and Laboratory Medicine. 2016;**54**(1):163-168. DOI: 10.1515/cclm-2015-0243

[107] Takahashi W, Nakada TA, Yazaki M, Oda S. Interleukin-6 levels act as a diagnostic marker for infection and a prognostic marker in patients with organ dysfunction in intensive care units. Shock. 2016;**46**(3):254-260. DOI: 10.1097/SHK.0000000000000616

[108] Bellos I, Fitrou G, Pergialiotis V, Thomakos N, Perrea DN, Daskalakis G. The diagnostic accuracy of presepsin in neonatal sepsis: A meta-analysis. European Journal of Pediatrics. 2018;**177**(5):625-632. DOI: 10.1007/s00431-018-3114-1

[109] Xiao T, Chen LP, Zhang LH, Lai FH, Zhang L, Qiu QF, et al. The clinical significance of sCD14-ST for blood biomarker in neonatal hematosepsis: A diagnostic accuracy study. Medicine (Baltimore). 2017;**96**(18):e6823. DOI: 10.1097/MD.0000000000006823

[110] Tabl HA, Abed NT. Diagnostic value of presepsin in neonatal sepsis. The Egyptian Journal of Immunology. 2016;**23**(2):29-37 PMID: 28502131

[111] Saied Osman A, Goudah Awadallah M, Tabl HAEL-M, TawfukAbed N, Saad S, Goudah E. Presepsin as a novel diagnostic marker in neonatal septicemia. Egypt Journal of Medical Microbiology. 2015;**24**(3):21-26

[112] Mostafa RM, Kholouss SM, MZakaria N, Hafiz TR, Abdelaziz DM. Detection of presepsin and surface CD14 as a biomarker for early diagnosis of neonatal sepsis. Journal of American Science. 2015;**11**(10):104-116

[113] Abdel Motalib T, Khalaf FA, El Hendawy G, Kotb SE, Ali AM, El Sharnoby A. Soluble CD14-subtype (Presepsin) and hepcidin as diagnostic and prognostic markers in early onset neonatal sepsis. Egyptian Journal of Medical Microbiology. 2015;**24**(3):45-52

[114] Ruan L, Chen GY, Liu Z, Zhao Y, Xu GY, Li SF, et al. The combination of procalcitonin and C-reactive protein or presepsin alone improves the accuracy of diagnosis of neonatal sepsis: A meta-analysis and systematic review. Critical Care. 2018;**22**(1):316. DOI: 10.1186/s13054-018-2236-1

[115] Kumar N, Dayal R, Singh P, Pathak S, Pooniya V, Goyal A, et al. A comparative evaluation of presepsin with procalcitonin and CRP in diagnosing neonatal sepsis. Indian Journal of Pediatrics. 2019;**86**(2):177-179. DOI: 10.1007/s12098-018-2659-3

[116] Parri N, Trippella G, Lisi C, De Martino M, Galli L, Chiappini E. Accuracy of presepsin in neonatal sepsis: Systematic review and meta-analysis. Expert Review of Anti-Infective Therapy. 2019;**17**(4):223-232. DOI: 10.1080/14787210.2019.1584037

[117] van Maldeghem I, Nusman CM, Visser DH. Soluble CD14 subtype (sCD14-ST) as biomarker in neonatal early-onset sepsis and late-onset sepsis: A systematic review and meta-analysis. BMC Immunology. 2019;**20**(1):17. DOI: 10.1186/s12865-019-0298-8

[118] Iskandar A, Arthamin MZ, Indriana K, Anshory M, Hur M, Di Somma S, et al. Comparison between presepsin and procalcitonin in early diagnosis of neonatal sepsis. The Journal of Maternal-Fetal & Neonatal Medicine. 2019;**32**(23):3903-3908. DOI: 10.1080/14767058.2018.1475643

[119] Poggi C, Lucenteforte E, Petri D, De Masi S, Dani C. Presepsin for the diagnosis of neonatal early-onset sepsis: A systematic review and meta-analysis. JAMA Pediatrics. 2022;**176**(8):750-758. DOI: 10.1001/jamapediatrics.2022.1647

[120] Kamel MM, Abd El Aziz RA, El Sayed MA, Abd-ullah HF. Presepsin as a predictor of positive blood culture in suspected neonatal sepsis. Malaysian Journal of Medical Research. 2019;**30**(4):138-142. DOI: 10.21608/mjmr.2022.221700

[121] Rashwan NI, Hassan MH, Mohey El-Deen ZM, Ahmed AE. Validity of biomarkers in screening for neonatal sepsis—A single center-hospital based study. Pediatrics and Neonatology. 2019;**60**(2):149-155. DOI: 10.1016/j.pedneo.2018.05.001

[122] Stojewska M, Behrendt J, Szymanska A, Pukas-Bochenek A, Stachurska A, Godula-Stuglik U, et al. Diagnostic value of presepsin (Scd14-St subtype): Evaluation in the detection of severe neonatal infections. International Journal of Research Studies in Biosciences. 2015;**1**(3):110-116

[123] Khater ES, Al-Hosiny TM. Presepsin as a new marker for early detection of neonatal sepsis in Al-Quwayiyah general hospital, Riyad, KSA. Journal of Advances in Microbiology. 2020;**21**(1):80-90. DOI: 10.9734/jamb/2020/v20i130210

[124] Zayed KM, Ali Saad AAE, Amin WM, El-Nasr MGA. Diagnostic value of presepsin in detection of early-onset neonatal sepsis. Al-Azhar Journal of Pediatrics. 2020;**23**(2):825-851. DOI: 10.21608/AZJP.2020.85889

[125] El-Madbouly AA, El Sehemawy AA, Eldesoky NA, Abd Elgalil HM, Ahmed AM. Utility of presepsin, soluble triggering receptor expressed on myeloid cells-1, and neutrophil CD64 for early detection of neonatal sepsis. Infection and Drug Resistance. 2019;**12**:311-319. DOI: 10.2147/IDR.S191533

[126] Ahmed AM, Mohammed AT, Bastawy S, Attalla HA, Yousef AA, Abdelrazek MS, et al. Serum biomarkers for the early detection of the early-onset neonatal sepsis: A single-center prospective study. Advances in Neonatal Care. 2019;**19**(5):E26-E32. DOI: 10.1097/ANC.0000000000000631

[127] Stoicescu SM, Mohora R, Luminos M, Merișescu M, Jugulete G, Năstase L. Presepsin-new marker of sepsis-Romanian neonatal intensive care unit experience. Revista de Chimie. 2019;**70**(8):3008-3013. DOI: 10.37358/RC.19.8.7475

[128] Yoon SH, Kim EH, Kim HY, Ahn JG. Presepsin as a diagnostic marker of

sepsis in children and adolescents: A systemic review and meta-analysis. BMC Infectious Diseases. 2019;**19**(1):760. DOI: 10.1186/s12879-019-4397-1

[129] Tanır Basaranoglu S, Karadag-Oncel E, Aykac K, Ozsurekci Y, Aycan AE, Cengiz AB, et al. Presepsin: A new marker of catheter related blood stream infections in pediatric patients. Journal of Infection and Chemotherapy. 2018;**24**(1):25-30. DOI: 10.1016/j.jiac.2017.08.012

[130] Baraka A, Zakaria M. Presepsin as a diagnostic marker of bacterial infections in febrile neutropenic pediatric patients with hematological malignancies. International Journal of Hematology. 2018;**108**(2):184-191. DOI: 10.1007/s12185-018-2447-x

[131] Fujii E, Fujino K, Eguchi Y. An evaluation of clinical inflammatory and coagulation markers in patients with sepsis: A pilot study. Acute Medicine & Surgery. 2019;**6**(2):158-164. DOI: 10.1002/ams2.397

[132] Shimoyama Y, Umegaki O, Kadono N, Minami T. Presepsin values predict septic acute kidney injury, acute respiratory distress syndrome, disseminated intravascular coagulation, and shock. Shock. 2021;**55**(4):501-506. DOI: 10.1097/SHK.0000000000001664

[133] Shimoyama Y, Umegaki O, Kadono N, Minami T. Presepsin values and prognostic nutritional index predict mortality in intensive care unit patients with sepsis: A pilot study. BMC Research Notes. 2021;**14**(1):245. DOI: 10.1186/s13104-021-05659-9

[134] Hassan EA, Abdel Rehim AS, Ahmed AO, Abdullahtif H, Attia A. Clinical value of presepsin in comparison to hsCRP as a monitoring and early prognostic marker for sepsis in critically ill patients. Medicina (Kaunas, Lithuania). 2019;**55**(2):36. DOI: 10.3390/medicina55020036

[135] Kim H, Hur M, Moon HW, Yun YM, Di Somma S, GREAT Network. Multi-marker approach using procalcitonin, presepsin, galectin-3, and soluble suppression of tumorigenicity 2 for the prediction of mortality in sepsis. Annals of Intensive Care. 2017;**7**(1):27. DOI: 10.1186/s13613-017-0252-y

[136] Drăgoescu AN, Pădureanu V, Stănculescu AD, Chiuțu LC, Florescu DN, Gheonea IA, et al. Presepsin as a potential prognostic marker for sepsis according to actual practice guidelines. Journal of Personalized Medicine. 2020;**11**(1):2. DOI: 10.3390/jpm11010002

[137] Matera G, Quirino A, Peronace C, Settembre P, Marano V, Loria MT, et al. Soluble CD14 subtype-a new biomarker in predicting the outcome of critically ill septic patients. The American Journal of the Medical Sciences. 2017;**353**(6):543-551. DOI: 10.1016/j.amjms.2017.03.036

[138] Jovanović B, Djurić O, Lj M-D, Isaković A, Doklestić K, Stanković S, et al. Prognostic value of presepsin (soluble CD14-ST) in diagnosis of ventilator-associated pneumonia and sepsis in trauma patients. Vojnosanitetski Pregled. 2018;**75**(10):968-977. DOI: 10.2298/VSP161104027J

[139] Masson S, Caironi P, Spanuth E, Thomae R, Panigada M, Sangiorgi G, et al. ALBIOS study investigators. Presepsin (soluble CD14 subtype) and procalcitonin levels for mortality prediction in sepsis: Data from the albumin Italian outcome Sepsis trial. Critical Care. 2014;**18**(1):R6. DOI: 10.1186/cc13183

[140] Wen MY, Huang LQ, Yang F, Ye JK, Cai GX, Li XS, et al. Presepsin

level in predicting patients' in-hospital mortality from sepsis under sepsis-3 criteria. Therapeutics and Clinical Risk Management. 2019;**15**:733-739. DOI: 10.2147/TCRM.S209710

[141] Zhao J, Tan Y, Wang L, Shi Y. Discriminatory ability and prognostic evaluation of presepsin for sepsis-related acute respiratory distress syndrome. Scientific Reports. 2020;**10**(1):9114. DOI: 10.1038/s41598-020-66121-7

[142] Aliu-Bejta A, Atelj A, Kurshumliu M, Dreshaj S, Baršić B. Presepsin values as markers of severity of sepsis. International Journal of Infectious Diseases. 2020;**95**:1-7. DOI: 10.1016/j.ijid.2020.03.057

[143] Popa TO, Cimpoeşu D, Dorobăț CM. Diagnostic and prognostic value of presepsin in the emergency department. Revista medico-chirurgicală a Societăţii de Medici şi Naturalişti din Iaşi. 2015;**119**(1):69-76 PMID: 25970945

[144] Brodska H, Valenta J, Pelinkova K, Stach Z, Sachl R, Balik M, et al. Diagnostic and prognostic value of presepsin vs. established biomarkers in critically ill patients with sepsis or systemic inflammatory response syndrome. Clinical Chemistry and Laboratory Medicine. 2018;**56**(4):658-668. DOI: 10.1515/cclm-2017-0839

[145] Koh JS, Kim YJ, Kang DH, Lee JE, Lee SI. Usefulness of presepsin in predicting the prognosis of patients with sepsis or septic shock: A retrospective cohort study. Yeungnam University Journal of Medicine. 2021;**38**(4):318-325. DOI: 10.12701/yujm.2021.01018

[146] EA TI, Eyrikh AR, Titova ZA. The role of presepsin in the diagnosis and assessment of severity of sepsis and severe pneumonia. Terapevticheskiĭ Arkhiv. 2018;**90**(11):44-47. DOI: 10.26442/terarkh2018901144-47

[147] Ugajin M, Matsuura Y, Matsuura K, Matsuura H. Impact of initial plasma presepsin level for clinical outcome in hospitalized patients with pneumonia. Journal of Thoracic Disease. 2019;**11**(4):1387-1396. DOI: 10.21037/jtd.2019.03.74

[148] Song X, Song Y, Yuan Y, Zhang P, Zhang X. Prognostic value of presepsin for outcomes and complications in enterocutaneous fistula complicated by abdominal sepsis. The International Journal of Surgery. 2016;**33**(Pt A):96-101. DOI: 10.1016/j.ijsu.2016.07.070

[149] Kim CH, Kim EY. Prediction of postoperative sepsis based on changes in presepsin levels of critically ill patients with acute kidney injury after abdominal surgery. Diagnostics (Basel). 2021;**11**(12):2321. DOI: 10.3390/diagnostics11122321

[150] Bamba Y, Moro H, Aoki N, Koizumi T, Ohshima Y, Watanabe S, et al. Increased presepsin levels are associated with the severity of fungal bloodstream infections. PLoS One. 2018;**13**(10):e0206089. DOI: 10.1371/journal.pone.0206089

[151] Xiao H, Wang G, Wang Y, Tan Z, Sun X, Zhou J, et al. Potential value of presepsin guidance in shortening antibiotic therapy in septic patients: A multicenter, prospective cohort trial. Shock. 2022;**57**(1):63-71. DOI: 10.1097/SHK.0000000000001870

[152] Yang HS, Hur M, Yi A, Kim H, Lee S, Kim SN. Prognostic value of presepsin in adult patients with sepsis: Systematic review and meta-analysis. PLoS One. 2018;**13**(1):e0191486. DOI: 10.1371/journal.pone.0191486

[153] Benovskaa M, Buckovaa D, Petrikova D, Stasek J, Gottwaldova J. Presepsin as a diagnostic and prognostic

tool for sepsis. Klinicka Biochemie a Metabolismus. 2015;**23**(3):89-94

[154] El-Shafie MES, Taema KM, El-Hallag MM, Kandeel AMA. Role of presepsin compared to C-reactive protein in sepsis diagnosis and prognostication. Egyptian Journal of Critical Care Medicine. 2017;**5**(1):1-12. DOI: 10.1016/j.ejccm.2017.02.001

[155] Yu H, Qi Z, Hang C, Fang Y, Shao R, Li C. Evaluating the value of dynamic procalcitonin and presepsin measurements for patients with severe sepsis. The American Journal of Emergency Medicine. 2017;**35**(6):835-841. DOI: 10.1016/j.ajem.2017.01.037

[156] Zhu Y, Li X, Guo P, Chen Y, Li J, Tao T. The accuracy assessment of presepsin (sCD14-ST) for mortality prediction in adult patients with sepsis and a head-to-head comparison to PCT: A meta-analysis. Therapeutics and Clinical Risk Management. 2019;**15**:741-753. DOI: 10.2147/TCRM.S198735

[157] Spanuth E, Ebelt H, Ivandic B, Werdan K. Diagnostic and prognostic value of soluble CD14 subtype (sCD14-ST) in emergency patients with early sepsis using the new assay PATHFAST presepsin. In: Proceedings of 21st International Congress of Clinical Chemistry and Laboratory Medicine, IFCC-WorldLab-EuroMedLab, Berlin, 15-19 May 2011. Clin Chem Lab Med. 2011;49(Suppl. 1):S361. doi: 10.1515/CCLM. 2011.066